1657

KU-710-335

ACEP Master Level Courses

ACEP Master Level courses are or will be available to accompany the following texts.

Sport Science

Coaches Guide to Sport Psychology by Rainer Martens discusses motivation, communication, leadership, and how to develop a variety of psychological skills.

Coaches Guide to Sport Physiology by Brian Sharkey leads coaches through the development of fitness-training programs suitable for their athletes.

Coaches Guide to Teaching Sport Skills by Robert Christina and Daniel Corcos uses practical examples to take coaches through the teaching/learning process.

Coaches Guide to Nutrition and Weight Control by Patricia Eisenman, Stephen Johnson, and Joan Benson provides practical guidelines to help coaches assist athletes in losing, gaining, or maintaining weight safely.

Coaches Guide to Social Issues in Sport by Jay Coakley and Robert Hughes examines how age, race, gender, and culture influence sport participation.

Coaches Guide to Sport Biomechanics describes the mechanical principles involved in sport movements.

Sports Medicine

Coaches Guide to Sport Injuries by J. David Bergeron and Holly Wilson Greene gives coaches information on injury prevention, emergency care, and follow-up procedures.

Coaches Guide to Sport Rehabilitation by Steven Tippett explains both the coach's role in rehabilitation and the process of rehabilitation as directed by health-care professionals.

Coaches Guide to Drugs and Sport by Bob Goldman examines the effects of a variety of abused drugs and the coach's role in combatting drug use.

Sport Management

Coaches Guide to Sport Law by Gary Nygaard and Thomas Boone explains the coach's legal duties in easy-to-understand terms.

Coaches Guide to Time Management by Charles Kozoll explains how to improve organization and avoid time-related stresses.

Coaches Guide to Sport Administration by Larry Leith provides guidelines to help coaches plan, organize, lead, and control their team's success.

Each course consists of a *Coaches Guide, Study Guide,* and *Workbook.* ACEP certification is awarded for successful course completion. For more information, please contact

ACEP
Box 5076
Champaign, IL 61825-5076
1-800-747-4457

Dedication

To Tina, Marissa, and Chris for your never-ending
understanding, patience, and support.

Contents

Preface   vii

Acknowledgments   ix

Part I: The Sport Rehabilitation Team   **1**

Chapter 1   The Coach   3
Chapter 2   The Physician   7
Chapter 3   Allied Health Specialists   11

Part II: Sport Rehabilitation Basics   **17**

Chapter 4   Sport Injury   19
Chapter 5   Sport Rehabilitation   31

Part III: Therapeutic Modalities of Sport Rehabilitation   **39**

Chapter 6   Modalities to Decrease Circulation   41
Chapter 7   Modalities to Increase Circulation   51
Chapter 8   Modalities to Decrease Pain and Inflammation   57

Part IV: Therapeutic Process of Sport Rehabilitation   **65**

Chapter 9   Exercises to Increase Range of Motion   67
Chapter 10   Exercises to Increase Muscle Strength   89
Chapter 11   Exercises to Improve Proprioception   105
Chapter 12   Protective Devices, Padding, and Supports   111
Chapter 13   Functional Progression: Returning to Activity   121

Appendix A   Stretching Reference   127
Appendix B   Therapeutic Exercise Reference   129
Appendix C   Functional Progression for Football   131
Appendix D   Functional Progression for Volleyball   137
Appendix E   Functional Progression for Baseball and Softball   141

Glossary   145

Suggested Reading List   149

Index   151

About the Author   157

Preface

As time winds down to under one minute left in the game, your star player twists an ankle and is unable to continue play. Your immediate concern for the athlete's well-being is somewhat eased as he or she gingerly limps off the court. But then you begin to wonder, How bad is the injury? Where should the athlete go for appropriate care? What can I do to speed up the rehabilitation process? When can I expect the player to return?

You have probably been in a similar situation and asked yourself similar questions. The purpose of the *Coaches Guide to Sport Rehabilitation* is to answer any question you may have regarding the rehabilitation process.

I will introduce you to the various members of the sports medicine team so you will better understand each professional's role in the injury management system. Specific guidelines regarding the coach's role during the recuperation period indicate how you can become an active participant in the rehabilitation process. Also, a background in general rehabilitation principles and their scientific bases will help you understand why certain rehabilitation techniques are better than others. Presented in a relevant, detailed, yet common-sense manner, this information will help you to better understand when your injured athletes will be ready to return to competition and the specific criteria they must meet before resuming full participation.

Every coach functions in a different environment as it relates to the care of the injured athlete. My goal in this book is to provide a common ground by establishing for you the following:

- A basis for interacting with the professionals involved in caring for your athletes
- A practical, working knowledge of the appropriate use of ice, heat, and compression and how these measures may help or in some cases hinder you in the rehabilitation process
- An understanding of therapeutic exercise methods designed to increase strength, flexibility, joint sense, and cardiovascular conditioning
- An awareness of special padding and bracing options available to the athlete that may allow them a safer and quicker return to competition
- An appreciation of your role in the especially crucial functional progression stage of rehabilitation, in which your athlete is tuning up for a return to game action

A coach informed in these basic areas of sport rehabilitation will be the best assistant to the attending sports medicine specialist and the injured athlete; so, all these areas are explored in detail in the *Coaches Guide to Sport Rehabilitation*. However, this book does not provide an in-depth analysis of every aspect of sport rehabilitation. Rather, it provides you with the practical knowledge required to assist in the sport rehabilitation process.

By working together and sharing their respective areas of expertise, coaches and sport rehabilitation professionals can attain their mutual goal of returning the athlete to competition safely and quickly and at the highest level of function possible.

Acknowledgments

Efforts to put the *Coaches Guide to Sport Rehabilitation* together required the assistance of some special people. Thanks first to the folks at Human Kinetics for allowing me to share my ideas on the appropriate care of injured athletes. Special thanks to Linda Bump and Ted Miller for the insight, structure, and expertise they provided. Also, without the efficient and prompt clerical help offered by Linda McIntire in preparing this book, I would still be fumbling at the keyboards. Finally, thanks are in order to you, the coach, for setting a constant example of dedication to the physical, personal, and social growth of the athlete.

PART I

The Sport Rehabilitation Team

Chapter 1
The Coach

It is only fitting to begin a resource for coaches on sport rehabilitation by examining the role you, the coach, should play as a member of the sport rehabilitation team. In fact, throughout the *Coaches Guide to Sport Rehabilitation* you will find suggestions as to how you can contribute to your athletes' rehabilitation.

Describing a role that applies to all coaches is virtually impossible, as every coach and coaching situation is unique. But in assuming a role in the rehabilitation of your athletes, you (and every coach) should consider

- your responsibilities as an emergency care provider;
- your limitations, legally and medically, in administering injury treatment; and
- your team's needs regarding a health care facility and staff.

THE COACH'S RESPONSIBILITIES IN PROVIDING INJURY CARE

As a coach who at times feels overburdened by the duties that accompany the job the last thing you want is additional responsibility. But, like it or not, as a member of the sport rehabilitation team you assume two more obligations:

- to stay informed of current sport rehabilitation principles and practices and
- to monitor the progress of each of your injured athletes during the rehabilitation process.

Stay Informed

A staggering number of sports medicine publications are now available that you should take advantage of to keep track of the latest methods in sport injury treatment and rehabilitation.

However, because sports medicine is in a boom period, the quality of material produced is sometimes questionable. And, even if the research is well conducted, it is frequently written in technical medical terms that are difficult to interpret.

Therefore, it is important that you have access to periodicals that provide current, accurate, and understandable sports medicine information. Here is a short list of publications that will help you fulfill your duty to stay informed.

Journals

Athletic Training (Greenville, NC: National Athletic Trainers' Association).

The First Aider (Gardner, KS: Cramer Products).

The Physician and Sportsmedicine (Minneapolis: McGraw-Hill).

Books

Booher, J.M., & Thibodeau, G.A. (Eds.) (1989). *Athletic injury assessment* (2nd ed.). St. Louis: C.V. Mosby.

Arnheim, D.D. (1984). *Modern principles of athletic training.* St. Louis: C.V. Mosby.

Roy, S.P., & Irvin, R.F. (1983). *Sport medicine: Prevention, evaluation, management, and rehabilitation* (6th ed.). Englewood Cliffs, NJ: Prentice-Hall.

In addition to reading, you should seek out experienced, qualified professionals who can answer your questions about sport injury rehabilitation. Athletic trainers, physical therapists, orthopedists, and others on the sports medicine team have devoted themselves to studying and applying methods of helping injured athletes return safely to activity. These individuals are usually pleased to help coaches who have a problem or concern.

If you are located in or near a metropolitan area, your local hospital is likely to have someone on staff who can either give you the information you need or provide the name, address, and phone number of an individual who can. If you live in a rural area, contact either a nearby hospital or a major university's sports medicine office. Many colleges have at least one team physician and several allied health professionals specializing in the care of athletes.

Monitor the Injured Athlete's Progress

In addition to staying informed of sports medicine principles and practices, you are responsible for staying abreast of the treatment and progress of your injured athletes. Three methods for doing so are

- communication,
- psychological and emotional evaluation, and
- physical observation.

Communication

An injured athlete often feels isolated from coaches and teammates. And, when an injury is severe and slow to heal, an athlete may no longer feel like part of the team. Withdrawal from the sport is common in such situations.

You can help an athlete stay involved as a team member throughout the healing and rehabilitation process by assigning the athlete duties such as keeping statistics, studying game films, or helping with scouting reports. Also, find time to visit with the athlete before or after practices and indicate your concern for his or her well-being. Communicate your concern for the athlete both as a person and as a contributor to the team.

Psychological and Emotional Evaluation

Although you probably don't have a degree in counseling or psychology, you should be sensitive to the mental and emotional strain experienced by injured players. Try to alleviate some of this tension by reassuring the athlete of his or her value to the team and emphasizing that the injury will not jeopardize future opportunities for participation.

It's normal for athletes to experience post-injury letdown. After all, something very important—athletic participation—has been stripped from them. On the other hand, most injuries are only temporary setbacks. So, help your athletes understand that the injuries they experience are simply short-term breaks in participation, not major catastrophes. Assure them that, if they follow the prescribed rehabilitation process, they probably will return to action quickly and safely.

Physical Observation

Although you should not diagnose injuries or their severity, you should frequently examine the healing progress of injuries that can be monitored visually. Sprained ankles, bruises, cuts, and other injuries may be inspected even by a medically untrained coach. If swelling increases or if signs of infection appear, you should have the athlete seen by a sports medicine specialist immediately.

Also, keep an eye on the athlete when he or she resumes activity. Are movements natural? Is the injured area favored in any way? Does the injured site swell following activity? Answer these questions satisfactorily before allowing an injured athlete to increase the intensity or duration of workouts.

THE COACH'S LIMITATIONS IN REHABILITATING INJURED ATHLETES

Although you, as a coach, can contribute much to the sport rehabilitation team, you also can severely threaten the rehabilitation process by overstepping your expertise. Specifically, you must be aware of your limitations in two areas:

- Legal
- Medical

Legal Limitations

Many states now require coaches to complete a first aid course and to be certified in administering cardiopulmonary resuscitation (CPR). Such requirements have led to a safer sport experience for millions of athletes and to the prevention of numerous potential tragedies.

However, coaches too often think they can identify an injury and recommend treatment, only to have the injury develop complications and threaten the career of an athlete. In fact, most sport injuries can be properly diagnosed and treated only by medical professionals and technologies.

If you allow previous experience or an unwarranted estimation of personal medical knowledge to recommend that an athlete not seek professional medical attention, you are setting yourself up for a losing legal battle. Or, if you return an athlete to activity before he or she is able to meet the demands of the sport, you could be held accountable.

Injury liability should be a concern of every coach, and no judge or jury will rule in favor of a coach who, with only rudimentary training, applies improper treatment or prevents an athlete from receiving prompt medical treatment.

Medical Limitations

If you're like most coaches, your medical training is limited or nonexistent. Perhaps you know how to tape an ankle or administer CPR but would probably be lost trying to distinguish between a dislocation and a subluxation (or the proper rehabilitation of the same). For example, if you've never tinkered with cars, you would be foolish to think that you could detect what was wrong with a car's engine, much less overhaul it.

Certainly, then, you would do well to learn more about sport injuries. Continuing education through ACEP's Sport First Aid and *Sport Injuries* (Bergeron, 1989; Bergeron & Greene, 1989) courses, courses offered by Cramer Products, and courses sponsored by a local college or sports medicine clinic represent valuable opportunities for coaches who are seeking more sports medicine knowledge. Additional training in advanced first aid is recommended and may be required if you are directly responsible for the care of your injured athletes.

You definitely should know emergency care and rehabilitation procedures. But, because of your limited experience in injury care, you must know who to turn to when athletes need medical assistance. So, let's look at some things you should consider when selecting health care assistance for your team.

THE COACH'S HEALTH CARE ASSISTANTS

The two components of health care are the *facility* in which care is provided and the *personnel* who administer the care. Both are important; and, as a coach who is responsible for seeing that your athletes get the best possible care, you should evaluate the medical facilities and their staffs in your area. Inquire specifically about the sports medicine equipment and staff, then follow up with a meeting and tour at the facility.

Perhaps you know other coaches in your area whose athletes are treated at various facilities. Ask their opinions of the service they have had and whether and why they would recommend the care providers they use.

As you evaluate these health care facilities, always keep in mind the particular needs of your athletes. In doing so, you should ask yourself whether the facilities and their staffs meet the "Four C" criterion:

- Convenient
- Comprehensive
- Competent
- Cooperative

Convenient

For practical purposes, your team's health care facility should be located close to the site of your practices and home competitions. This facility should be ready to respond to athletic injuries when they occur and should have sufficient treatment hours to meet the needs of your athletes during rehabilitation. Also, professionals at the facility should be available when your injured athletes have free time in their schedules.

Comprehensive

Your team's health care must be medically based. The technology used should be state of the art, and you should familiarize yourself with the equipment to understand its functions and limitations in treating your athletes.

The staff at the facility should not simply hide behind buttons and switches. They should provide full and logical explanations for using their therapies and be candid about their ability to treat and rehabilitate an athlete's injury.

Competent

Most professional groups have, or are working toward, certification requirements. Make sure you inquire about the certification status of your team's health care staff, that is, whether they were formally tested or whether certification was awarded simply by paying an annual fee.

Also, check your health care staff's experience. How many years have they been practicing their specialties? What is their track record? What kind of reputation do they have among other sports medicine professionals? What do other coaches say about the service they have received from the staff?

Once you are satisfied that the staff is properly certified and experienced, ask for references that you can contact to verify their expertise. Remember, you are placing a great deal of trust in their hands, so it is better to be thorough in the selection process than regretful after an injury was treated incompetently.

Cooperative

Many nearby health care facilities will have the equipment, the versatility, and the professional expertise to serve your team. Far fewer, however, are likely to share your philosophy or communicate in a manner you find satisfactory.

Many facilities foster dependency by en-couraging the athlete and coach to turn to them even when professional health care treatment is not warranted. Some facilities are unduly conservative and hold injured athletes out of competition long after a safe return was possible. Make certain that the health care facility you select shares your objective: to safely return the athlete to the highest level of function in the shortest time possible.

Part of your role involves communicating your concerns and receiving feedback about your athletes' injuries from the sports medicine specialists at the facility. Indeed, establishing rapport between you and the health care staff is essential if your athletes are to have a cohesive and effective sport rehabilitation team to serve them. And it's your duty to see that they do!

CHAPTER SUMMARY

1. You play a vital role in the rehabilitation of your injured athletes no matter what your experience or situation.
2. You have two major responsibilities in sport injury rehabilitation: to stay informed of the basic principles and practices in sport injury care and to monitor closely the progress of your injured athletes throughout the rehabilitation period.
3. You should be keenly aware of your legal and medical limitations in overseeing the care of injured athletes.
4. When selecting a health care facility and staff, you should consider whether they meet the Four C criterion: convenient, comprehensive, competent, and cooperative.

Chapter 2
The Physician

As mentioned in chapter 1, because of your medical and legal limitations, you should never assume the role of a health care professional. You should, however, be familiar with the sports medicine specialists who will be so important to the rehabilitation of your athletes and who will be your partners on the sport rehabilitation team. First, though, let's take a brief look at the sports medicine field in general.

THE FIELD OF SPORTS MEDICINE

Sports medicine is one of the fastest growing areas in health care. Medical and paramedical sport-related positions are now common throughout all levels of athletics, in hospitals and clinics, at fitness centers, and within corporations. Students are flocking to the field in record numbers as a result of the increasing popularity of sport, the health-and-fitness craze, and the opportunity to work with highly motivated athletes in a meaningful, professional manner.

In this book, two major categories of sports medicine specialists are examined. In this chapter you will read about the training, role, and areas of expertise of a sport physician. In chapter 3 you will be introduced to the allied health specialists in sport: the athletic trainer, the physical therapist, the dietician, the physiologist, the psychologist, and the strength and conditioning coach.

THE ROLE OF A SPORTS MEDICINE SPECIALIST

Sports medicine has so many subspecialties because each facet of the athlete's readiness to compete must be fine tuned for optimal performance. In the case of the injured athlete, each component of health and fitness must be addressed before he or she can return safely to competition. It is impossible for one person to obtain the knowledge and training necessary to be competent in all these specialized areas of sports medicine. Therefore, sports medicine and, in particular, sport rehabilitation require a team approach.

When these sports medicine specialists combine their efforts, a comprehensive system of athlete care is formed. Among the wide range of duties they provide are the following:

- They *educate* athletes and coaches about risks, precautions, and treatments.
- They *prevent* injury and reinjury by instituting training regimens and safety measures.
- They *treat* injuries by using the most appropriate methods.
- They *rehabilitate* the injured athlete as quickly as possible to full function.

THE SPORTS MEDICINE PHYSICIAN

Many sport organizations have a team physician, that is, a doctor with a specific interest and training in sports medicine. Such individuals are invaluable to a coach because they combine a thorough understanding of medicine's injury diagnoses and treatments with a knowledge of sport's physiological demands and risks. Therefore, when a team physician is available, you should consult him or her before making any significant health care decision involving a player on your team.

Physicians practicing sports medicine have completed 4 years of undergraduate study, 4 years of medical school, and from 2 to 6 years of a residency program. They often choose to specialize in a particular area of medicine and emphasize this training in their sports medicine practice. As you will see, sports medicine physicians come from a wide array of these specialized fields.

Types of Sports Medicine Physicians

The diversity of specializations among physicians practicing sports medicine makes imperative the establishment of treatment standards and quality control. Fortunately, several sports medicine groups are both instituting mechanisms for ensuring competency and conducting evaluations of team physicians. For example, the American Academy of Sports Physicians has established a written examination that physicians may take to demonstrate sports medicine expertise.

As you examine the qualifications of a sports medicine physician, you also should determine which type of physician would be best for your athletes. As you read about the following three most common types of sports medicine physicians, consider which injuries occur most often in your sport and what the medical needs of your athletes might be:

- Pediatrician
- General practitioner
- Orthopedist

Pediatrician

The pediatrician is a physician who specializes in the care of children and often is the youth-sport athlete's first contact with the medical system.

General Practitioner

The family practice physician typically cares for adolescent athletes when a pediatrician is not available or not utilized. Adult amateur and recreational athletes are also frequently seen by the general practitioner.

Orthopedist

The orthopedist is perhaps most responsible for the tremendous evolution in sports medicine during the past 10 to 15 years, mainly because of the types of injuries one is trained to treat. The orthopedist specializes in evaluat-

ing, classifying, and treating disorders of the musculoskeletal system (muscles and bones) and related structures (ligaments, cartilage, and tendons).

Additional Types of Sports Medicine Physicians

Although the pediatrician, general practitioner, and orthopedist are the most common types of sports medicine physicians, doctors with specialized training in other areas of medicine also may care for athletes. Depending on the type of injury experienced by an athlete, you might consider contacting a sports medicine physician who specializes as one of the following:

- Cardiologist
- Dentist
- Dermatologist
- Neurologist
- Neurosurgeon
- Ophthalmologist
- Oral surgeon
- Otolaryngologist
- Podiatrist

Cardiologist

A cardiologist may be consulted to evaluate and treat any circulatory and heart conditions or exercise tolerance difficulties experienced by your athletes.

Dentist

Routine preventive and maintenance care of teeth are the most common ways in which the dentist assists athletes. But the dentist should also be visited by athletes who have displaced or fractured teeth, problems with the temporal-mandibular joints (jaws), or other emergency problems involving the mouth.

Dermatologist

A dermatologist should be consulted by athletes having problems with the largest organ of the body—the skin.

Neurologist

A neurologist must be contacted for head or neck injuries. This specialist manages disorders of the central nervous system (brain and spinal cord) and the peripheral nervous system (nerves in the legs, arms, and trunk).

Neurosurgeon

A neurosurgeon is a neurologist who also has the expertise to perform surgical procedures. Therefore, one should be called on to intervene in serious injuries to the central and peripheral nervous systems.

Ophthalmologist

If an athlete suffers an injury to an eye or its surrounding structures, an ophthalmologist (and perhaps an optometrist) should be consulted.

Oral Surgeon

A dentist with surgical training—an oral surgeon—should be used to treat serious problems that arise in and around the mouth.

Otolaryngologist

An otolaryngologist (or ear-nose-throat specialist) can treat conditions involving an athlete's mouth, ears, nose, and throat and is often consulted when surgical intervention is needed for facial fractures.

Podiatrist

Athletes experiencing problems of the feet, ankles, or lower legs should see a podiatrist for care. In addition, a podiatrist can provide orthotics (custom-made shoe inserts) to treat poor foot alignment and structure.

CHAPTER SUMMARY

1. Sports medicine is a growing health care field that is also increasing in sophistication and specialization.
2. The expertise of sports medicine specialists includes the ability to educate, prevent, treat, and rehabilitate athletes.
3. Sports medicine physicians are well-trained medical experts who also have knowledge of sport and the effects of physical activity on the athlete's body.
4. The three most common types of sports medicine physicians are pediatricians, general practitioners, and orthopedists.
5. Other specialized physicians who may practice sports medicine include cardiologists, dentists, dermatologists, neurologists, neurosurgeons, ophthalmologists, oral surgeons, otolaryngologists, and podiatrists.

Chapter 3
Allied Health Specialists

The increased specialization and delineation of roles within sport has led to even more specialization in the allied health professions. These specialists aren't physicians but are nonetheless valuable members of the sport rehabilitation team. Their areas of expertise span from the physical to the mental aspects of athletic performance. Thus, you can utilize allied health professionals as a group or individually to provide comprehensive or specific assistance. Among the allied health specialists available to you are the following:

- Athletic trainer
- Physical therapist
- Dietician
- Exercise physiologist
- Sport psychologist
- Strength and conditioning coach

ATHLETIC TRAINER

Athletic training is the profession that has been dedicated the longest to the care of athletes. Because of the knowledge and the techniques the profession has developed over time, a qualified athletic trainer can be a tremendous asset to you. These highly dedicated professionals work countless hours behind the scenes to help you and your athletes in many ways.

Duties and Responsibilities

Athletic trainers demonstrate knowledge and skill in prevention and care of athletic injuries, acute management of injury, fitting of protective padding and equipment, taping, bandaging, and other areas of sports medicine.

Certified athletic trainers work with high school, college, and professional athletes. They are also involved with amateur sport groups, ranging from individual sport federations to Olympic and national teams.

Specific duties of the athletic trainer in the rehabilitation process include acute injury assessment and management of acute situations. When employed in an educational setting, the trainer also oversees formal rehabilitation of the athletes from that school. Clinic trainers assist with the rehabilitation efforts of athletic injuries referred for treatment by appropriate medical personnel. As sports medicine clinics grow in number, so does the number of trainers working at these centers.

Whether working in an educational setting, an amateur training center, or a clinic, the trainer must be directly supervised by a medical doctor. Formal interaction with the team or independent physician treating an athlete is required.

Although athletic trainers are licensed in some states, services provided by the trainer are not reimbursed by third-party payers (i.e., insurance companies). At the collegiate or professional level, liability issues are of less concern because the trainer functions under the guidance of the team physician and treats only athletes from that particular institution or organization. This is also true at the high school level if the trainer is employed by the school. Clinic-based trainers work under the direct supervision of the referring physician or a physical therapist if one is employed by the clinic.

Education and Training

Qualified trainers in sports medicine are certified. A certified athletic trainer, or ATC, has completed at least a 4-year undergraduate program of study consisting of coaching, physical education, and the basic sciences as they relate to the care of the athlete. Some trainers opt to continue schooling, taking courses toward a Master of Science degree that provide more specialized training in the sciences and in the use of exercise and treatment modalities. After completing formal education, the trainer must pass the written, oral, and practical parts of a national examination. This examination process and the schools offering a training curriculum are approved by the National Athletic Trainers' Association, an organization founded in the early 1950s. Several states have instituted athletic trainer practice acts that require the trainer to be licensed.

PHYSICAL THERAPIST

The field of physical therapy is extremely popular today. Numerous job opportunities are available in the many different areas of physical therapy, including sports. However, confusion often arises when discussing the role of the physical therapist (PT), especially when comparing it to that of athletic trainer.

Duties and Responsibilities

In sports, the PT is usually based in a clinic that may be affiliated with a hospital or a physician's office or that may be an independent agency.

Physical therapists are closely involved in the care of the athlete after injury has occurred, designing and implementing rehabilitation programs to return the athlete to participation. In many states it is legal for a PT to evaluate a patient without the order of a physician. Some states also allow evaluation and treatment without physician referral, whereas many do not allow any hands-on treatment without physician orders. Physical therapy services are routinely reimbursed by third-party coverage.

Education and Training

Physical therapists complete a minimum of 4 years of formal training that emphasizes basic and advanced sciences as they relate to the treatment of physical disability. Postgraduate work in physical therapy usually focuses on a specialized area at the master's or doctoral level. Basic education covers foundations for the evaluation and treatment of musculoskeletal, neurological, cardiopulmonary, and other conditions.

Physical therapists who want to become more proficient in sport may attempt to become certified as athletic trainers. However, this may no longer be necessary as the physical therapy profession has moved into the area of specialization. Sports physical therapy is 1 of 17 sections of the American Physical Therapy Association. Many of the 17 sections, including sports physical therapy, offer examinations to certify a PT as a specialist in a given area. The sports physical therapist must have at least 5 years of experience in the field of rehabilitation before taking the certification examination.

Physical therapists must pass a written examination in the state where they desire to practice as a licensed professional. Some states also require the successful completion of an oral examination.

DIETICIAN

Allied health care professionals who are trained specifically in the field of nutrition are called dieticians. An athlete's performance can be enhanced with the aid of sound nutrition, and the dietician is the resident expert in this field. For example, during the rehabilitation process, the dietician may be consulted when an athlete is being treated for a psychological problem in the form of an eating disorder. Athletes being rehabilitated for physical problems may also exhibit nutritional problems that the dietician may assist in managing.

Duties and Responsibilities

Most dieticians are employed by a hospital. Often, they serve as consultants to athletes and teams on dietary matters. The dieticians' areas of expertise in sport include weight gain and loss, bulimia, anorexia nervosa, precompetition meals, proper hydration, and nutritional supplementation.

Education and Training

This professional has a college degree in dietetics. Dieticians interested in sports medicine belong to the Sports and Cardiovascular Practice Group, the largest special interest group with the American Dietetic Association.

EXERCISE PHYSIOLOGIST

Physiology is the study of how the human body functions. General human physiology examines such body functions as digestion, respiration, and circulation. As science has become more specialized, however, so too has the study of physiology.

Exercise physiologists are interested in the heart, lungs, muscles, endocrine and exocrine glands, and other structures that function both during and after exercise. An exercise physiologist may be consulted to study an athlete's level of exercise fitness before, during, or after sport participation. Research conducted by the exercise physiologist can help answer questions related to an athlete's tolerance to a rehabilitation program.

Duties and Responsibilities

Exercise physiologists holding doctoral degrees are often based at universities where they conduct research, teach, or both. Exercise physiologists at the master's level may also work in academic settings, or they may design and run exercise programs in hospitals, health clubs, or corporate industries.

Education and Training

Exercise physiologists usually have at least a master's degree in their areas of specialization, and, as the field becomes more complex and

competitive, completion of a doctoral degree is common. These professionals often belong to the American College of Sports Medicine (ACSM), which was organized in 1954 and has pioneered the growth of exercise science. Special certification in areas of exercise related to cardiac conditioning and general rehabilitation is available through the ACSM. Membership in this group transcends the area of exercise physiology as members of many other professions also belong to the ACSM.

SPORT PSYCHOLOGIST

A psychologist is a trained professional in the area of psychology but differs from his or her medical counterpart, the psychiatrist, in that the psychologist need not be a medical doctor. A sport psychologist differs from a psychologist in that the former devotes most of his or her practice to athletes and is rarely state licensed.

Sport psychology in the United States has developed quickly since the mid 1960s. Now, many universities have at least one sport psychologist on faculty, and teams and athletes commonly employ sport psychologists as assistant coaches or consultants.

Duties and Responsibilities

Sport psychologists at a university conduct research and assist athletes in a variety of ways. The sport psychologist helps athletes learn how to maximize their performance by using principles of psychology as they relate to sport. Applied sport psychologists emphasize enhancing sport performance through mental skill training that involves such skills as positive thinking, motivation, relaxation, stress management, and imagery.

Education and Training

The sport psychologist has completed a 4-year course of undergraduate studies with postgraduate studies at the master's level and usually at the doctoral level. The field of sport psychology is working toward developing an accreditation program. Two groups to which sport psychologists typically belong are the Association for the Advancement of Applied Sport Psychology and the North American Society for Psychology of Sport and Physical Activity.

STRENGTH AND CONDITIONING COACH

As strength is a vital component of sport, the individual trained in building athletic strength is an important member of the sport rehabilitation team.

Duties and Responsibilities

Strength and conditioning coaches typically are employed by college and professional football programs, but other levels of football and other sports may also hire or consult a strength-training coach. The professional strength-training coach provides expertise in the proper utilization of strength-training apparatus, strengthening programs for the specific muscles important for a given sport, efficient and safe movement patterns for common strength-training programs, and individualized in-season and off-season conditioning programs. Strength-training coaches are also able to explain specific movement patterns and the biomechanics of common sports activities, ranging from swimming the breaststroke to hitting a hockey slap shot. The strength-training coach helps the athlete to maximize muscular performance by sport-specific strengthening and to prevent injury by using proper lifting techniques.

Education and Training

Although the strength-training coach is not technically a health care specialist, many of them who are certified are trained as health care specialists such as athletic trainers or physical therapists. On the other hand, many certified strength coaches are members of coaching staffs and have no formal health care background. Certified strength coaches have passed a national certification examination devised in conjunction with the National Strength and Conditioning Association.

CONTACTING ALLIED HEALTH SPECIALISTS

Do not hesitate to contact any of the following allied health organizations for more information. They will be happy to help you.

American College of Sports Medicine (ACSM), PO Box 1440, Indianapolis, IN 46206

American Physical Therapy Association (APTA), 1111 N. Fairfax St., Alexandria, VA 22314

Association for the Advancement of Applied Sport Psychology (AAASP), University of North Carolina, Department of Physical Education, CB #8605, 315 Woollen, Chapel Hill, NC 27599

National Athletic Trainers' Association (NATA), 1001 E. Fourth St., Greenville, NC 27858

National Strength and Conditioning Association (NSCA), PO Box 81410, Lincoln, NE 68501

CHAPTER SUMMARY

1. Nonphysicians that are often involved in the care of the athlete are the athletic trainer, the physical therapist, the dietician, the exercise physiologist, the sport psychologist, and the strength and conditioning coach.
2. Each of these health care specialists plays a unique role on the sports medicine team. You should be familiar with their respective roles to utilize each team member appropriately.

Part Summary

This part of the *Coaches Guide to Sport Rehabilitation* described your role and the roles of others on the sport rehabilitation team. Much of the responsibility is yours, so you should seek out qualified and cooperative sports medicine specialists to share in the rehabilitation phase. After reading Part I, you should have an idea of who these specialists are, their qualifications and areas of expertise, and how they can help you in your role as an informed supervisor of quality care for your athletes during rehabilitation.

PART II

Sport Rehabilitation Basics

Chapter 4
Sport Injury

In this part we examine the basics of sport rehabilitation. An understanding of these principles is necessary if you are to contribute effectively to the rehabilitation effort.

In this chapter, the components of a rehabilitation program and the goals of rehabilitation for sport injury are presented. These topics are not addressed in depth, so you should not attempt to design a sport rehabilitation program from the knowledge you gain in this part. Rather, in this chapter and chapter 5, you will gain a more thorough understanding of how to deal with your injured athletes and learn how to work with the appropriate sports medicine specialists. The basics presented here and the specifics that follow should enable you to do both.

DEFINING AND DIAGNOSING SPORT INJURIES

Before you can fully appreciate the importance of sport rehabilitation, you must first understand sport injury. To assist in a program to help your athletes get better, you must be able to determine what's wrong. Without knowing the mechanisms of injury (how the athlete is injured), how injuries are classified, the typical responses of involved tissue to injury, and other injury-related issues, you cannot begin to understand the process of sport rehabilitation. So let's look first at the things that can go wrong—sport injuries—and then discuss how you can have a positive effect on the athlete after injury occurs.

Defining Sport Injury

Because there are so many types of injuries, I limit my discussion of things that can go wrong with the athlete to those conditions arising from injuries sustained in sport. My focus is narrowed further to injuries involving muscles, tendons, bones, ligaments, and other tissues of the musculoskeletal system as most injuries sustained in sport involve these structures.

Other body structures and systems are less frequently injured but are also treated by members of the sports medicine team. Injuries to such areas are mentioned when appropriate but are not dealt with in great detail. Common illnesses experienced by athletes also are beyond the scope of this book.

Diagnosing Sport Injury

A sound sport rehabilitation program begins with an accurate diagnosis of the injury. The evaluation of an injured athlete should be timely, comprehensive, and correct. The sports medicine specialist's evaluation skills are developed only through proper education and experience.

You are only flirting with disaster if you attempt to evaluate and then single-handedly manage a particular injury. However, an informed, trained coach can assist in the identification of a sport injury. Such a coach knows his or her athletes and when their movements are not normal. This insight can be very helpful to the physician in the early diagnosis of overuse injuries or other medical conditions.

Regardless of one's training or intuition, however, a prudent coach will limit his or her diagnostic role to referring the athlete for appropriate medical assessment. Whether the condition involves the musculoskeletal, cardiovascular, neurological, or other body system, proper assessment must be performed by the appropriate professional.

OVERUSE VERSUS ACUTE INJURY

Injuries, or trauma, to the musculoskeletal system of the athlete can be classified as acute (macrotrauma) or as related to overuse (microtrauma).

Macrotrauma

Macrotrauma is an acute injury in which a single traumatic event causes injury to a previously healthy structure, for example, when a healthy athlete falls on the point of a shoulder and sustains an acromioclavicular sprain (separated shoulder). Other examples of macrotrauma follow:

- Acute fracture
- Dislocation and subluxation
- Sprain and strain
- Contusion
- Laceration
- Abrasion

An *acute fracture* can result when bone encounters high-impact forces that commonly result from falls, collisions, or excessive twisting.

A *dislocation* occurs when the continuity of a joint is disrupted. In other words, because of a previous traumatic event, the bones making up the joint may no longer provide the support to maintain joint integrity. Joints that are frequently dislocated in sport are those of the shoulder (glenohumeral); the patella, or kneecap (patellofemoral); and the fingers (metacarpal-phalangeal or interphalangeal) (see Figure 4.1).

Subluxation can occur acutely when the force of a movement is not quite sufficient to produce a dislocation. Restraints to abnormal motion at the joint are stretched, but the joint still maintains continuity. These so-called minidislocations are also common at the shoulder (glenohumeral) and patellar (patellofemoral) joints.

Sprains are injuries to ligaments and are usually classified according to the amount of laxity present (see Table 4.1).

Strains are injuries to muscle tissues or tendons. The classification of muscle strains is shown in Table 4.2.

Additional acute macrotrauma commonly sustained in sport are contusions, lacerations, and abrasions.

Table 4.1
Classification of Ligament Sprain

Classification	Degree of fiber disruption	Amount of laxity
First degree (mild)	None	None
Second degree (moderate)	Minimal to moderate	Moderate, but with a stopping point
Third degree (severe)	Total	Severe, with no stopping point

Table 4.2
Classification of Muscle Strain

Classification	Degree of fiber disruption	Joint status
First degree (mild)	None	Painful, but no weakness; full range of motion
Second degree (moderate)	Minimal to moderate	Limited range of motion; weak and painful passive stretch
Third degree (severe)	Total	Significantly decreased active motion; painful passive stretch

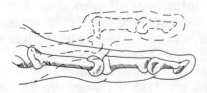

Figure 4.1. Finger dislocation (proximal interphalangeal joint).

Microtrauma

Microtrauma refers to an overuse injury. Unlike macrotrauma, the resultant injury is caused not by a one-time event but by cumulative events. Microtrauma results from repetitive, submaximal loading on a body structure, whether it be pitch after pitch, rebound after rebound, or stroke after stroke. These repetitive, sport-specific actions produce stress on a given bone or soft tissue. When forces associated with a movement tear down tissue at a greater rate than nature can regenerate it, bone and soft tissue break down.

Although specific examples of microtrauma are described later, a few common forms of overuse injuries are

- tendinitis,
- traction apophysitis,
- bursitis, and
- stress fracture.

Tendinitis, or inflammation of a muscle tendon, often affects the upper extremities of swimmers and throwers and the lower extremities of runners and jumpers.

Common forms of *traction apophysitis* experienced by growing athletes are Osgood-Schlatter's disease and Sever's disease. Both are prompted by adolescent growth spurts, in which muscles pull excessively on small bumps of bone that are trying to fuse to larger bones. Osgood-Schlatter's disease involves the tibial tubercle trying to fuse to the tibia (the larger of the lower leg bones), whereas Sever's disease involves the tibial tubercle trying to fuse to the calcaneous (heelbone). This pulling action prevents the tubercles from fusing to the larger bones, producing inflammation and pain at the site.

A small fluid-filled sac called a *bursa* decreases friction at critical sites in the musculoskeletal system. Chronic friction at a given area may result in *bursitis* (inflammation of the bursa). Common anatomical areas of bursitis in sport are the shoulder (subacromial bursa), elbow (olecranon bursa), and around the knee (prepatellar and pes anserine bursas).

Stress fractures are occurring with greater frequency and at earlier ages than ever before. Lower extremity stress fractures are frequently seen in runners, dancers, and jumpers but can be found in any athlete involved in a sport requiring prolonged, stressful weight bearing.

Gymnasts also experience stress fractures in both the upper extremity (wrist and elbow) and the lower back.

Other bone problems that are thought to be due, in part, to overuse and excessive loading involve injury to the joint surface. *Osteochondritis dissecans*, or OCD, is a common condition of the joint surface of the ankle, knee, or elbow. Another bone-stress-failure reaction occurs at the end of the clavicle (collarbone) and often results from excessive bench pressing.

ANATOMY OF AN INJURY

Many excellent textbooks describe athletic injury in detail. They typically classify injury by body part and then describe the structures involved, how these structures are injured, and what is generally done to rehabilitate the injury.

This book, however, specifically addresses sport rehabilitation. Therefore, the descriptions of sport injuries and of the structures involved in those injuries are brief. And, because the injuries discussed are organized by anatomical area, a brief review of anatomy is included within each of the following sections.

Head and Neck Injuries

Athletic injuries involving the head and neck usually occur in contact or collision sports such as football, hockey, lacrosse, and rugby. However, athletes in any sport involving frequent and forceful contact with an opposing player or playing surface are vulnerable to head and neck injuries.

The injuries discussed in this section specifically involve the seven cervical vertebrae and the accompanying spinal nerves (see Figure 4.2).

The nerves of the cervical area branch off the spinal cord, one to the right and one to the left, and then exit small holes (intervertebral foramen) located between two cervical vertebrae. Cervical nerves are named according to their relationship with the cervical vertebrae. For example, the nerve that exits between the base of the skull and the first cervical vertebra is referred to as C-1 (first cervical nerve); C-2 (second cervical nerve) exists between the first and the second cervical vertebrae and so on.

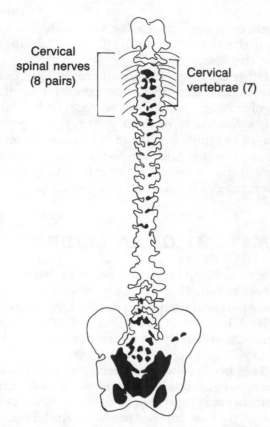

Figure 4.2. Seven cervical vertebrae and the accompanying spinal nerve roots exiting from each side.

Cervical spinal nerves (8 pairs)

Cervical vertebrae (7)

Brachial Plexus Stretch

A frequent injury in contact sports involving the cervical nerves is a *brachial plexus stretch*, also known as a *stinger* or *burner*. *Plexus* is a term used to describe a group of nerves. In this case, the brachial plexus refers to five nerves in the neck region, that is, C-5 to T-1 (first thoracic nerve).

A stinger results when the head is laterally flexed to one side as the shoulder on the opposite side is lowered. A common mechanism for the injury is a tackle in football. As the neck is laterally flexed to the right and the left shoulder depressed, the brachial plexus on the left is stretched. Stretching the affected nerves results in a sharp buzzing or stinging sensation down the affected arm, hence the name "stinger." Recurrent brachial plexus stretches may result in permanent nerve damage.

Sprains and Strains

The muscles and ligaments of the cervical spine can be strained or sprained as a result of many sport activities. Muscles involved in such injuries can be superficial (lying close under the skin) or deep (lying underneath the superficial muscles) (see Figure 4.3a and b).

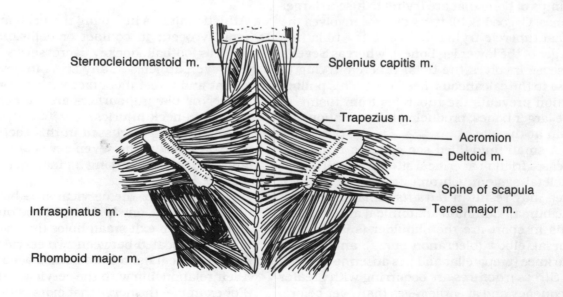

Sternocleidomastoid m.

Splenius capitis m.

Trapezius m.

Acromion

Deltoid m.

Spine of scapula

Teres major m.

Infraspinatus m.

Rhomboid major m.

a

Figure 4.3a. Superficial muscles of the cervical spine.

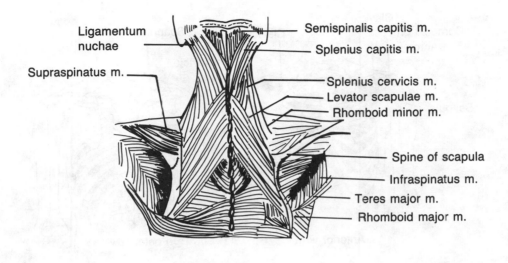

Figure 4.3b. Deep muscles of the cervical spine.

Upper Extremity Injuries

The upper extremities are subjected to a wide variety of stresses in many sports and thus are susceptible to a wide variety of sport injuries. The upper extremities include the humerus (upper arm bone), the radius and the ulna (bones of the forearm), the eight carpal bones (wrist bones), and the metacarpals and phalanges (hand and finger bones, respectively) (see Figure 4.4).

Also included, but often forgotten, is the shoulder girdle complex, a function of which is to connect the arm to the body. The bones that constitute the shoulder girdle are the scapula (shoulder blade) and the clavicle (collarbone) (see Figure 4.5).

Because the upper extremity must be freely mobile, tremendous stresses are placed on the joints and muscles that allow this freedom of movement as they simultaneously protect it from excessive or abnormal motion. These stresses often lead to acute or chronic sprains and strains.

Impingement Syndrome

Impingement syndrome is an overuse shoulder injury often sustained by athletes who perform repetitive overhead motions. Baseball pitchers, volleyball spikers, and freestyle swimmers are the most frequent victims.

The mechanism of impingement syndrome involves the supraspinatus tendon of the rotator cuff, the biceps tendon, or both being pinched between the humerus and the coracoacromial ligament (see Figure 4.6). The space between the humerus and the ligament is narrow. Thus, repetitive overhead motions may cause tendon irritation and subsequent inflammation. When the tendon becomes inflamed, it enlarges and takes up even more of the already limited space. The thicker the tendon is, the more easily it is pinched; and the more the tendon is pinched, the thicker it becomes. Chronic shoulder pain, decreased strength, and subpar athletic performance result.

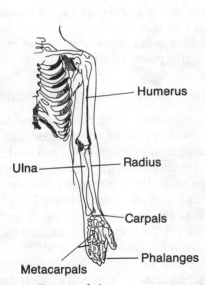

Figure 4.4. Bones of the upper extremity.

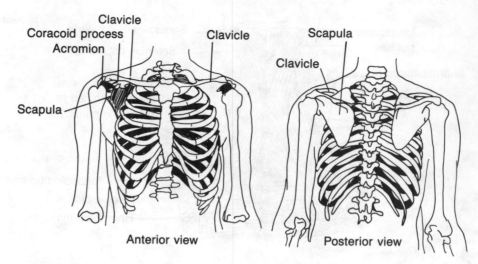

Figure 4.5. Bones of the shoulder girdle.

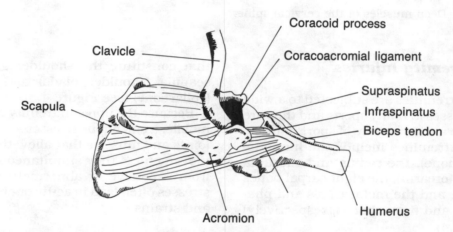

Figure 4.6. Impingement syndrome. As the arm is lifted overhead, the supraspinatus and/or biceps tendon is pinched between the humerus and the coracoacromial ligament (superior view).

Shoulder Dislocation

Shoulder dislocation most frequently occurs with the humerus directed anteriorly (forward) out of the glenoid cavity. When the shoulder becomes dislocated, its primary restraint to abnormal motion, the joint capsule, is damaged.

Common mechanisms of anterior shoulder dislocation are a fall on an outstretched arm, a blow to the back of the shoulder, or a force applied to the arm or forearm with the shoulder out to the side (abducted).

Acromioclavicular Sprain, or Shoulder Separation

Another common injury sustained in sports, the separated shoulder, is a sprain of the liga-

ments attaching the clavicle to the acromion process (tip of the shoulder).

Shoulder separations most often result from falls on the point of the shoulder.

Lateral and Medial Epicondylitis

Lateral epicondylitis, better known as "tennis elbow," is one of the most difficult sport injuries to rehabilitate. Involved in this injury are the tendinous origin of the wrist extensors and two muscles specifically involved at the lateral epicondyle: the extensor carpi radialis brevis and the extensor digitorum communis (see Figure 4.7). Pain can typically remain for a year in chronic cases, well after normal strength and flexibility have returned.

Epicondylitis is typically seen in racket sports, and possible reasons for its develop-

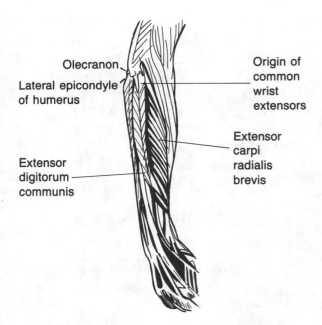

Figure 4.7. Muscles of the lateral epicondyle.

ment are improper technique (usually a faulty backhand), inadequate muscle flexibility or strength, and improper equipment (poor racket construction or string tension). *Medial epicondylitis* involves the tendinous origin of the wrist and finger flexors.

Another common condition involving the medial elbow is *medial elbow overload*. This condition frequently strikes athletes during the acceleration phase of throwing. It is then, as the athlete brings the arm forcefully forward to throw, that ligaments on the medial side of the elbow are stressed.

Common precipitating events leading to medial overload are inadequate warm-up, trying to throw too hard, and improper throwing mechanics.

The shoulder and elbow injuries previously described are but a few of the common sport injuries affecting the upper extremities. However, let's move on now to some of the injuries most frequently afflicting the lower extremities.

Lower Extremity Injuries

Running, jumping, hopping, and kicking are but a few of the activities required in most sports. The adequate function of the lower extremities is a vital prerequisite and is often taken for granted by athletes and coaches until injury occurs.

The bones of the lower extremity are the femur (thigh bone), patella (knee cap), the tibia and fibula (lower leg bones), the seven tarsals (bones constituting the ankle) and the metatarsals and phalanges (foot and toe bones, respectively) (see Figure 4.8).

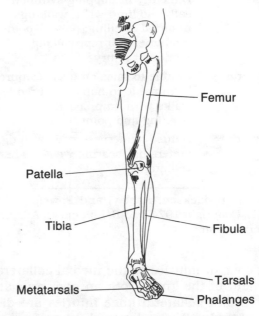

Figure 4.8. Bones of the lower extremity.

Joints frequently involved in lower extremity sport injury are the hip, where the femur joins the pelvis at the acetabulum (hip socket); the knee joint, where the femur and the tibia join; and the ankle joint, where the tibia and fibula form the talus. Another joint that causes many lower extremity problems is the patellofemoral joint, which is comprised of the femur and the patella.

Sprains

Sprains to the ligaments of the lower extremity are the most frequently reported injuries in all sports at all levels.

Ankle sprains occur with great frequency, one of the most common mechanisms being one athlete stepping on the foot of another (for a practical grading system for ankle sprains, see Table 4.3).

Knee sprains are increasing in frequency and occurring at younger ages. Not surprisingly, then, one of the hottest topics of discussion in sports medicine today is the proper management of anterior cruciate ligament sprains of the knee. Rule changes restricting blocking below the waist in football have reduced the

Table 4.3
Functional Classification of Ankle Sprain

Classification	Ankle status and function
Mild	Difficulty in hopping symmetrically; no limp when walking; minimal swelling; pain or point tenderness on reproducing motion of injury
Moderate	Unable to raise on toes of injured leg; unable to hop on injured leg; walks with limp; localized swelling and point tenderness
Severe	Diffuse tenderness and swelling; prefers not bearing weight when walking

Note. From Jackson, Ashley, and Powell (1974, p. 201). Copyright 1974 by J.B. Lippincott. Adapted by permission.

incidence of injuries to the medial collateral ligament of the knee. Both anterior cruciate and medial collateral knee injuries are discussed in detail later in this book.

Strains

Strains involving muscles of the lower extremity are also common. Muscle groups frequently involved are the groin (hip flexors and adductors), hamstrings, and quadriceps. Contributing factors to lower-extremity muscle strains are imbalanced muscle strength, inadequate muscle flexibility, and improper training technique (inadequate warm-up, improper stretching, etc.).

Tendinitis

Tendinitis is a chronic inflammation of a muscle tendon, most often involving the iliopsoas (hip flexor muscle), the patellar and Achilles tendons, and the iliotibial band (see Figure 4.9). I discuss these conditions in greater detail when I describe specific exercises used to stretch (chapter 9) and strengthen (chapter 10) these structures to decrease the likelihood of their being injured.

Plantar Fasciitis

The plantar fascia is a tough, fibrous band that runs along the bottom of the foot and offers

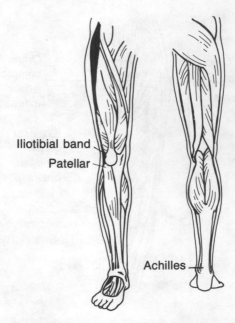

Figure 4.9. Common sites of lower extremity tendinitis: a, patellar tendon; b, iliopsoas tendon; c, achilles tendon; d, iliotibial band.

support to the foot's arch. The structure can become chronically inflamed. Athletes with abnormal foot structure may be predisposed to *plantar fasciitis.*

TISSUE RESPONSE TO INJURY

Now that you have a general overview of sport injuries you need to understand what actually happens to body tissue when it is injured. Swelling results when the degree of injury is sufficient to produce a break in the continuity of local blood flow.

Causes of Swelling

Normally, fluid mechanics and pressures keep fluid within the circulatory system. However, when the smallest blood vessels (capillaries) are injured, the fluid contained within the vessels escapes. The area that the fluid escapes to is an empty space called *interstitial space* (or extracellular space).

Cells damaged by sport injury or by being inadequately nourished through decreased circulation will die. Cell death causes a release of histamine, which in turn causes the blood vessels to dilate, thus bringing more fluid to an area poorly equipped to handle it. This excess fluid produces swelling.

Healing Effects of Swelling

Although this extra fluid slows down the rehabilitation process, it plays a necessary part in healing. Chemicals (histamine, serotonin, and bradykinin) present at the injury site produce local inflammation and pain.

Local inflammation, characterized by warmth, redness, and pain, allows more blood to enter the area. This inflammation and an accompanying increase in blood flow permit easier fluid exchange between the vessel wall and the interstitial space. This activity enhances the local cleanup of dead cells and promotes healing.

Thus, as you will clearly see when I discuss the modalities used to decrease swelling, it is difficult to regulate the local fluid mechanics that help resolve the injury without compounding the damage further.

Pain-Spasm-Ischemia Cycle

Pain is experienced for many reasons. Local damage to tissue can cause painful nerve fiber irritation. Pain also arises from excess fluid exerting pressure on sensitive nerve endings. A breakdown in circulation to an injured area or a restriction of blood flow both to and from an injured site also produces pain.

Pain causes local skeletal and smooth muscle to spasm voluntarily or involuntarily. Muscle spasm further compromises local blood flow (ischemia), yielding yet more pain. It is difficult to intervene in this vicious pain-spasm-ischemia cycle once it is established. Properly administered therapeutic modalities and exercise can help. And the "PRICE" injury management system, which I will soon discuss, is effective in decreasing the effects of acute injury.

POSTINJURY PHASES

The goals of sport rehabilitation and the treatment programs used to accomplish these goals vary, depending on the phase the injury is in.

An injury can be divided into the

- acute phase,
- subacute phase, and
- chronic phase.

Acute Phase

The *acute phase* of sport injury refers to the immediate 48 to 72 hours after the injury occurs. This phase is characterized by pain, swelling, muscle weakness, and decreased range of motion. Although these symptoms of acute injury are a nuisance, they are vital in allowing the body to resolve the injury.

Subacute Phase

After the acute phase ends, the *subacute phase* begins. During this phase, swelling and pain begin to subside, and muscle strength and joint motion increase; the emphasis now is on regaining normal use of the injured body part. The subacute phase ends when the athlete has regained full motion and normal muscle strength and experiences no swelling or pain during athletic activity.

Chronic Phase

The *chronic phase* is the period 6 months after the initial injury. Chronic injury can be defined as those conditions resulting in reinjury or as unresolved injuries resulting in swelling, pain, or the residual loss of motion or strength.

INTERVENING IN SPORT INJURY

The use of many components in the management of sport injury is dictated by the athlete's response to specific intervention. For example, in the course of returning the athlete to play, function must be smooth, unrestricted, and automatic. If the athlete cannot perform without a compromise in function, then a return to play should be delayed until full function is restored. Therefore, reevaluation of the athlete's condition, progress, and tolerance to activity is constantly required. These are the areas in which you can utilize your knowledge in assisting in the rehabilitation effort.

PRICE Management of Acute Injury

Perhaps you learned the acronym PRICE when it used to be ICE or RICE. (It seems that another letter is added every year or so.) Nevertheless, this management system for acute injury should be employed as soon as possible after injury occurs. Because you are often present at the scene of an injury, your expediency in implementing the PRICE principles will help your athlete return to competition more quickly.

P—Protection | Refrain from all painful positions and activities for at least 48 hours. Crutches, slings, splints, and so on may be required for pain-free activity.

R—Rest | All activity causing increased discomfort or swelling should be avoided. Motions that do not produce pain at an injured joint, as well as motion at uninjured joints, should be encouraged.

I—Ice | Apply ice to an injured area until it is numb (20 to 30 minutes) every 2 hours. When icing a joint, remove the ice every 4 to 5 minutes and move the joint gently.

C—Compression | Utilize intermittent or continuous compression after removing ice or use compression in conjunction with ice. See that proper pressure and wrapping techniques are used.

E—Elevation | Elevate the involved body part above the heart. Incorporate pain-free active range of motion with elevation.

Treating Overuse Injuries

Chronic overuse injuries respond to therapeutic exercises and modalities. These overuse syndromes are categorized according to the degree and occurrence of pain. Specifically, you may find the modified Blazina system helpful in determining whether an athlete's injury is getting better or worse (see Table 4.4).

Table 4.4
Modified Blazina Staging

Injury level	Degree of pain	Effect of pain on performance
1	No pain	None
2	Pain with extreme exertion that disappears when activity stops	None
3	Pain with exertion, remaining 1-2 h after exertion	Hinders performance
4	Pain during athletic activity, remaining 4-6 h after exertion	Pain worsens with activity; performance negatively affected
5	Pain starting as soon as athletic activity begins	Removal from that activity
6	Pain with activities of daily living	Prevents sport performance

Note. From Curwin and Stanish (1984, p. 101). Copyright 1984 by Sandra Curwin and William D. Stanish. Adapted by permission.

The Coach's Role

Your role in the management of chronic injury is to recognize the level of the injury and modify your athletes' activities accordingly. In managing acute problems, you should follow the PRICE program, be able to apply standard first aid care, render appropriate emergency care within the limits of your training, and know how to activate the emergency medical system (EMS).

But don't stop there; read further and learn more so you'll be a much better informed and more able member of the sport rehabilitation team. The chapters that follow provide greater detail regarding the therapeutic means (exercises and modalities) used to safely and quickly return injured athletes to competition. Also presented are other, perhaps more coach-oriented components of sport rehabilitation, such as protective padding and functional progression.

CHAPTER SUMMARY

1. You must understand sport injury before you can take an active role in the rehabilitation process.
2. Sport injury can be roughly categorized as macrotrauma or microtrauma. Macrotrauma is characterized by a single traumatic injury event. Microtrauma refers to injury resulting from repetitive movements that result in injury.
3. The demands of a given sport activity make certain macrotraumatic events or microtraumatic episodes more or less likely. Long-distance runners, for example, are frequently victims of microtrauma, whereas sprinters more often succumb to macrotrauma.
4. Knowledge of the inherent demands of a given sport activity, a sound medical background, and adequate clinical skills are required for accurate assessment of athletic injury. As a coach, you should defer injury diagnoses to medical professionals.
5. The body's response to injury is a natural physiological process. The clinical signs of this response (pain, swelling, inflammation, ischemia, etc.) must be treated in the sport rehabilitation process.
6. You should know how to implement the PRICE management system to treat acute injuries. And you should know how to classify overuse injuries and appropriately modify activity to prevent the injury from becoming worse.

Chapter 5

Sport Rehabilitation

With a general overview of sport injury behind us, we can now concentrate on the process of restoring the injured body part to full function. But before I discuss the rehabilitation process in depth, you should be introduced to the components of sport rehabilitation.

COMPONENTS OF A SPORT REHABILITATION PROGRAM

Every sport rehabilitation program should include the following:

- Prevention
- Assessment
- Goal setting
- Implementation
- Reevaluation

Prevention

The old sayings that an ounce of prevention is worth a pound of cure and that the best treatment is prevention certainly apply to sport rehabilitation. I explain this important component in great detail later in this chapter.

Assessment

Before initiating a rehabilitation program, you must know the nature and extent of the condition being rehabilitated. As discussed previously, it is *not your role to diagnose* any injury. If the performance of your athlete is compromised because of an injury, then it is safe to say that injury assessment and subsequent rehabilitation are in order.

In the case of acute injury, you should implement the PRICE injury management system. Acute injury resulting in a compromise of the athlete's airway, breathing, or circulatory status requires you to perform emergency measures for which you should be trained. In the case of overuse injury, you should be able to classify the stage of injury and act appropriately.

You can also assist in the management of your athletes' injuries by helping to determine how injuries happened. The diagnosis of a sport injury is much easier when the athlete or someone who witnessed the injury is able to accurately describe how the injury occurred. If you witnessed the injury, your accurate description of the incident can be especially beneficial to the attending sports medicine specialist.

Goal Setting

After accurately assessing an injury, you should help in setting treatment goals. The goals you set should be realistic and based on the problem areas discovered during the assessment.

Goals are often classified as short term or long term. Short-term goals are those that are attainable in a period of days to weeks. Long-term goals are those that are attainable after the completion of the short-term goals and are usually expressed in periods of weeks or longer.

Implementation

A rehabilitation program can be designed and implemented only after you and medical professionals have evaluated the problem, looked for deficiencies (ways in which the athlete's condition differs from normal), and subsequently devised goals for returning the injured part to normal.

Reevaluation

Once the rehabilitation program has been designed and is being carried out, the athlete's tolerance to the program must be monitored continuously. The best rehabilitation program is one that stresses your athlete to the maximum but is not detrimental to rehabilitation.

Applying the Components of Sport Rehabilitation

Perhaps the components of rehabilitation can be best described by an example. A forward on your basketball team comes down from a rebound onto another player's foot. The athlete limps off the court and takes the shoe and sock off the injured limb. Already you notice swelling.

You have the athlete elevate the foot, and ice is applied over the swollen area. You do not let the athlete return to the game. After the game the athlete is X-rayed; the test is negative for fracture. Your team physician now orders rehabilitation for the athlete's ankle sprain.

So far, you have assessed the injury and taken appropriate steps for acute injury. Now the rehabilitation specialist will perform a baseline assessment of the athlete and establish treatment goals. Short-term goals are established to manage pain and swelling and to increase range of motion and strength. Long-term goals are set to return the athlete to competition when pain and swelling are gone and range of motion and strength reestablished.

Once the goals have been set, appropriate means to accomplish these goals are chosen by the rehabilitation specialist.

After the rehabilitation program has been implemented, your athlete's tolerance to the program is monitored by the specialist with your assistance. When the treatment program's goals have been accomplished, the athlete is allowed to return to competition.

GOALS OF A SPORT REHABILITATION PROGRAM

Any sport rehabilitation program you institute with an athlete should be guided by these three goals:

Goal #1: Preventing injury

Goal #2: Restoring optimum function

Goal #3: Returning the athlete to competition quickly and safely

Goal #1: Preventing Injury

The first goal in sport rehabilitation is prevention. Most athletic training curricula offer courses in the care and prevention of athletic injury. Areas to be considered in efforts to prevent injury include

- adequate safety measures,
- proper training methods, and
- preseason screening.

Adequate Safety Measures

Ensuring adequate safety for your athletes is your ultimate responsibility. As a coach, it is your duty to see that all necessary equipment required for the sport is of satisfactory quality and is repaired properly and maintained well. The condition of the playing field or playing environment is also your responsibility. This includes (but is not limited to) maintaining indoor and outdoor playing surfaces, providing adequate protective padding and barriers, controlling indoor temperature regulation, allowing appropriate outdoor activities on the basis of environmental conditions, and adhering to rules governing your sport.

Proper Training Methods

Just as it is your duty to ensure that the playing surfaces are suited for safe competition, even more important is your responsibility to make certain that your athletes are physically suited for the sport. Your athletes should have strong minds and bodies and be ready to accept the demands of the sport. You need to make sure that adequate strengthening and stretching programs are offered to the athlete, that off-season and in-season cardiovascular work is performed, and that sound nutritional practices are used. You should not forget that the athlete is a person, so you also have the responsibility to provide for the personal and social growth of your athlete not only with teammates but also as a student and a member of society.

Preseason Screening

Preseason screening programs are another way of preventing injury. Adequate, thorough preparticipation physical examinations are a vital prerequisite for all athletes. As a coach you should confirm that the physicals have been completed and establish rapport with those responsible for performing the physical exam. If you find that the physicals are not being performed or that the paperwork is simply being pushed through, take steps to correct the situation; for, if a condition arises that should have been caught in the preparticipation physical, you can be just as liable as the physician who supposedly performed the exam.

The preparticipation exam, in addition to a standard medical checkup, should also include a sport-specific, comprehensive musculoskeletal evaluation. Ideally, these exams should be performed far in advance of the season so that any deficiencies discovered can be addressed. Body areas at risk in a given sport should be given special attention. Flexibility, strength, joint stability, coordination, endurance, and any other related aspects should be carefully evaluated. Previously injured or problem areas may warrant special testing or continual follow-ups.

Goal #2: Restoring Optimum Function

No matter how comprehensive a screening mechanism is and how conscientious the efforts of you and the medical team are, injuries can still happen. When they do occur, athletes should receive prompt and qualified medical attention and evaluation. A treatment plan for the injured athlete should then be formulated with attainable short- and long-term goals for recovery and rehabilitation. The athlete, coach, and sports medicine team should all be aware of the specific treatment goals and the methods to be employed to attain the goals.

Goals of the sport rehabilitation effort are multifaceted but can be summarized generally as those means used to *safely return the injured athlete to the highest level of function in the shortest time possible*:

- Decrease pain and swelling
- Normalize strength, endurance, and flexibility
- Restore proprioception
- Reestablish aerobic and anaerobic fitness
- Recover sport-specific function

Decrease Pain and Swelling

Pain is the body's way of telling you that something is not quite right. Pain and swelling that occur as a result of sport injury must be controlled immediately after injury. As you will see in Part III, there are means available to help you address these problems.

Normalize Strength, Endurance, and Flexibility

Strength.   Muscle function is required to produce joint movement. The human body moves in a sophisticated fashion, assuming the positions and performing the tasks required for sport. And muscles are the prime movers that allow athletes to move in this fashion. Muscles also provide dynamic stability to joints, aid in respiration, and carry out automatic functions routinely taken for granted (e.g., blinking the eyes).

When injury to a muscle occurs, the muscle tissue is less capable of generating force because of muscle fiber damage. In addition, pain from the injury causes reflex muscle shutdown (reflex inhibition). And immobilization renders a muscle weak, causing it to assume an abnormal resting length.

Athletic rehabilitation, therefore, must include activities to normalize muscle strength, length, and endurance. Exercises must be specific enough to isolate involved structures to maximize strengthening and stretching efforts but not so specific that all the stress is placed on only the involved muscle or muscle group. This is especially important because muscle balance must be restored as well. Muscles acting on one side of a joint can become weaker or stronger than those on the opposite side of the joint.

A good example is the ratio between the strength of the quadriceps and hamstring muscles. Commonly, athletes do much quadriceps strength training in such activities as squats, leg presses, knee extensions, and sled work. Conversely, the hamstrings are rarely the focus of strength-training activities. And, even if they were, these muscle are more difficult to work than the quadriceps because there are fewer hamstring-strengthening methods available. The normal ratio between hamstring and quadriceps strength is 60% to 70%. That is, the hamstrings are usually 60% to 70% as strong as the quadriceps. However, muscular athletes commonly have hamstring-to-quadriceps ratios from 35% to 45%. Among the clinical implications of this muscle imbalance are high risks for initial and recurrent hamstring strains (especially in athletes involved in sprinting).

Endurance. Once an injured athlete's muscle strength has approached normal and a normal resting muscle length is present, your rehabilitation efforts should be directed toward reestablishing muscle endurance through high-repetition, low-resistance activities. Methods to address inadequate muscle length and strength are discussed in chapters 9 and 10.

Flexibility. Swelling, decreased muscle strength, immobilization, and injury to structures within a joint can restrict normal joint motion. Range of motion (ROM) is important in

- maintaining extensibility of soft tissue,
- maintaining nourishment of articular cartilage (cartilage lining the bones that make up a joint), and
- allowing muscle to exert maximal force.

Thus, you can see, restrictions in ROM can lead to decreased flexibility, poorly nourished articular cartilage, and decreased muscle strength.

Deficiencies in muscle length can be corrected by balancing each side of a particular joint to allow full excursion of the muscle and full joint motion. The knee, for example, must be balanced on each side of the joint. Walking, running, and many other activities require slight flexion of the knee. But, because we spend many of our waking hours in seated

positions, hamstring muscle length is not frequently stressed to the end of the motion (complete knee extension) (see Figure 5.1). Therefore, this important muscle group is often shorter than the complementary quadriceps group, and a muscle imbalance results at the knee.

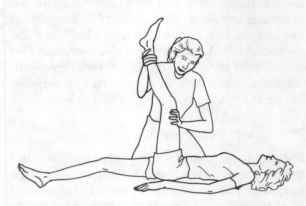

Figure 5.1. Assessing hamstring flexibility. With the athlete supine, bend the hip to a 90° angle and ask the athlete to straighten the knee. The knee should actively straighten to less than 10° from a completely straight position.

Some degree of hamstring tightness is inherent in everyone unless the hamstrings are routinely stretched. Also, the calf muscles are rarely stressed to maximum length in routine activities and so are also tight in many individuals unless an organized effort to stretch the calves is routinely performed.

Tight hamstrings and calves create greater resting tension on structures on the opposite side of the knee. The example I like to use is a bow and arrow. The further the bowstring is pulled back, the more stress is placed on the bow. Likewise, the tighter the hamstrings and the calves, the greater the resting tension on the front of the knee. Also, the tighter the calves and hamstrings, the harder the quadriceps must work to overcome the resistance of the calves and hamstrings. The greater the quadriceps force, the greater the pull on the extensor mechanism (quadriceps tendon, patella, patellar tendon, and tibial tubercle).

Clinical implications of inflexible hamstring and calf muscles are a greater incidence of patellofemoral pain, jumper's knee, patellar tendinitis, Osgood-Schlatter's disease, and other knee-related problems. Full, unrestricted joint ROM attained by proper stretching thus both protects the joint from excessive forces and facilitates optimal body-part movement. Screening mechanisms to assess muscle length are presented in chapter 9.

Keep in mind that the normal ROM for a nonathlete may not be normal for an athlete in a given sport. For example, normal active external rotation of the shoulder is 0° through 90° (see Figure 5.2a). However, active rotation for a baseball pitcher is approximately 130° to 150° (see Figure 5.2b). Therefore, a ROM of 130° to 150° is not normal for a nonthrowing athlete but is vital for a high-caliber baseball pitcher. It then follows that a pitcher would not be allowed to participate until normal ROM had been reestablished.

Restore Proprioception

For an athlete to perfect a sport skill, a certain sequence of events must occur. You must first introduce and demonstrate the skill to the athlete, who must then practice the new skill. Then, feedback as to the correctness of the athlete's performance must be given to the athlete, who must then use the feedback and repeatedly practice the skill until it becomes more or less automatic.

Athletes must go through a similar learning process after joint injury or immobilization. Injured tissue must be "reinstructed" to do what is correct. The human body's feedback loop is made possible by *proprioception*, which is the ability of a joint to tell the brain where that joint is in space. This feedback loop must be operational so that the muscle can act on a given joint to correct the joint's position after the joint tells the brain what that position is

and the brain tells the muscle to fire. Activities to reinforce joint sense are required before coordinated muscle function can be achieved.

Reestablish Aerobic and Anaerobic Fitness

When an athlete is recuperating from an injury, the period of rest that is required to allow healing may be prolonged. Prolonged downtime can produce substantial deconditioning. The following are a few of the many physiological effects of deconditioning:

- Muscle weakness
- Disuse muscle atrophy
- Immobilization osteoporosis
- Decreased cardiovascular conditioning
- Decreased lung capacity

Activity should be resumed as soon as possible during the rehabilitation period to prevent the detrimental effects of inactivity. If aerobic and anaerobic training can continue during rehabilitation, the athlete's return to competition will be quicker.

Aerobic fitness. Aerobic refers to the body's utilization of oxygen to produce energy. An aerobic base is necessary for both aerobic and anaerobic sport activities. To maximize training for aerobic cardiovascular fitness, athletes should work out for at least 20 to 30 minutes three times a week at a heart rate 65% of their predicted maximum rate.

Calculating a Training Heart Rate

A variety of methods can be used to determine an effective aerobic training heart rate, the

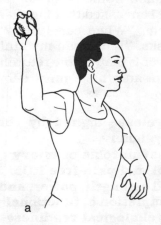
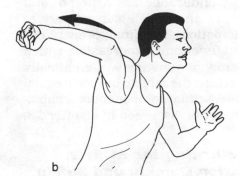

Figure 5.2. External rotation of the shoulder: a, normal external rotation for a nonthrowing athlete (about 90°); b, normal external rotation for a baseball pitcher (130° to 150°).

most accurate being a graded exercise stress test on a treadmill. However, a simpler way is to instruct your athletes to subtract their age from 220. Then, have them multiply that number (their predicted maximum heart rate) by .65. For example, a 17-year-old athlete would subtract 17 from 220 to get 203 beats per minute as the maximum predicted heart rate. To train aerobically, the athlete should elevate the heart rate 65% of 203, or 132 beats per minute, and keep it there for at least 20 to 30 minutes.

When lower extremities are injured, athletes can focus their training on upper extremity fitness. For lower extremity injuries, pool running can be performed in the deep end of a pool by using a flotation jacket for support when no weight is to be placed on the affected leg. The athlete who is able to bear weight may run in the shallow end of the pool. With some lower extremity injuries, cycling on a stationary bike may be allowed. Upper extremity injuries will almost always allow such cycling activity and possibly jogging or running.

Anaerobic fitness. Anaerobic fitness is often overlooked in sport rehabilitation. Many sports are primarily anaerobic, yet preseason screening, training, and rehabilitation programs often fail to take into account anaerobic function. Sprinting, interval training, quick bursts on a bike or an upper extremity ergometer, line jumping, and step-ups are among the activities that may be incorporated into the rehabilitation program for sport-specific durations.

Recover Sport-Specific Function

When an injured area demonstrates full ROM with no pain, strength and muscle endurance are back to normal, proprioception and aerobic and anaerobic endurance are restored, and swelling is gone, the athlete can prepare to resume participation. This final, preparatory phase is called *functional progression*, which refers to a series of activities systematically organized to return the athlete to sport-related function. This essential component of rehabilitation is thoroughly discussed in chapter 13.

Goal #3: Returning the Athlete to Competition Quickly and Safely

The previously mentioned components of rehabilitation deal primarily with the first goal of sport rehabilitation: returning the athlete to the highest level of function possible. Now let's talk briefly about the second goal of sport rehabilitation: safely returning the athlete to his or her sport in the shortest time possible.

Time Frames for Resuming Participation

Time frames to accomplish this goal are just that—time frames—in that every situation is unique. Bone usually takes 4 to 8 weeks to heal, some longer, and yet some fractures never heal. Others take less than 4 weeks before protected participation is allowed.

Sprains and strains usually heal in 4 to 6 weeks; however, longer periods of time may be required, depending on the tissue involved and the degree of severity.

Soft-tissue injuries must be given adequate time to heal. Although pain, swelling, strength, motion, and function usually are the primary considerations, other factors must be taken into account before allowing an athlete to resume playing.

When to Say It's OK to Play

There are no hard-and-fast rules for deciding when an injured athlete can return to participation. Every athlete and every injury is different. Therefore, each injury should be evaluated on an individual basis, with no preset time frames or norms for returning to participation. Moreover, every situation is unique. For example, a senior high school athlete playing his last-ever football game might be allowed to compete, whereas if the same injury had occurred a year earlier or if the athlete has a chance to play college football the next year, participation would be discouraged.

When I am asked that familiar question by an athlete, "When can I play?" or when a coach asks, "When can my athlete return?" my answer is that, before returning to full participation, an athlete must demonstrate the following:

- **A release signed by the attending physician**
- **No symptoms of injury**
- **Full and pain-free ROM**
- **Full strength, power, and endurance**
- **Completion of functional progression**
- **Psychological readiness**

Once the athlete is ready to resume participation, he or she may also need additional bracing, padding, and support to decrease the likelihood of reinjury. This important part of sport rehabilitation is addressed in detail in chapter 12.

The sport rehabilitation program is a complex process. The basics presented in this chapter are discussed in more detail in the following chapters.

CHAPTER SUMMARY

1. The first goal of sport rehabilitation is to prevent sport injuries. Many methods to decrease the likelihood of injury can be instituted by you, the coach.

2. Components of a sport rehabilitation program also include assessment, goal setting, implementation, and re-evaluation.

3. Other goals of sport rehabilitation include restoring optimum function and returning the athlete to competition as quickly and safely as possible.

4. For an athlete to return to competition, he or she must first show a release signed by the attending physician; no symptoms of injury; full and pain-free ROM; full strength, power, and endurance; completion of functional progression; and psychological readiness.

Part Summary

Before one can begin to thoroughly understand a given subject, the basics of that subject must be comprehended. This part presented the basics of sport injury and the fundamentals of sport rehabilitation. Also presented were ways in which you can help prevent sport injury and the criteria for allowing your athletes to return to competition after injury. A good grasp of these sport rehabilitation guidelines, of how an athlete is injured, and of what happens to the body after injury will help you better handle your injured athletes.

PART III
Therapeutic Modalities of Sport Rehabilitation

Modalities, as discussed in this chapter, are the particular machines and physical means the sports medicine specialist uses in caring for athletes. Heat, cold, pressure, and electrical stimulation are a few of the modalities used in rehabilitation. Ice, hot packs, and ultrasound are common therapeutic means by which these modalities are delivered to the injured athlete. It is important that you comprehend how and why these measures are critical for the rehabilitation of your athletes.

Certain pieces of therapeutic equipment are absolutely necessary in the care of today's athlete, whereas others are not always needed. I don't rate every piece of equipment that's available on the market, but I do examine the various uses of a particular modality, describe what that modality does, and identify its potential benefits.

Most modalities are used to break up the pain-spasm-ischemia cycle that was discussed in chapter 4. I present and then categorize the various treatment modalities by their desired physiological effects. Specific attention is given to the effects of these modalities on circulation, pain, and inflammation.

Although you may not perform many of the treatments described, you should be aware of the *precautions* and *contraindications* that are discussed for each modality. If you identify any of these precautions or contraindications, you should immediately report them to the sports medicine specialist performing the treatment.

Chapter 6
Modalities to Decrease Circulation

Excess fluid (swelling) in an injured body part impedes circulation and prolongs the healing process. As was discussed in chapter 4, swelling can be a major problem immediately after soft-tissue injury. Management of acute soft-tissue injury often requires the use of methods to decrease circulation and thereby decrease swelling.

The two most common modalities used to decrease local blood flow to minimize swelling are cryotherapy (cold therapy) and external compression. Some modes of electrical stimulation are used to manage swelling as well. In this chapter, I describe these three modalities for reducing swelling. But first, let's examine what these modalities are used to treat: swelling.

THE PHYSIOLOGY OF SWELLING

To understand how ice and other means (i.e., high-voltage galvanic stimulation and compression) to decrease swelling work, you must first understand where swelling comes from.

All living tissues in the body are nourished by oxygen carried through the circulatory system. Vessels carrying oxygenated blood away from the heart are, in order from largest to smallest, the aorta, the arteries, the arterioles, and the capillaries. The wall of a capillary is a one-cell-thick layer that permits the ready exchange of water, oxygen, and other molecules to nourish cells of the body. The area between the unicellular cell wall and the cells to be nourished is called the interstitial (or extracellular) space.

Normal Local Circulation

In normal fluid mechanics, the local circulatory system is in balance, being maintained largely by the role of proteins found in blood plasma. Normally, the protein concentration of the blood plasma located in the capillary is approximately four times that of the blood plasma located in the interstitial space. This is because the pores between the capillary wall and the interstitial space are narrower than the plasma proteins. Small amounts of the proteins do pass through the pores in normal situations, but these very small amounts return to the circulatory system by way of the *lymphatic system*, the body's filtering system, and then return to the heart by way of the *venous system*.

Overstimulated Local Circulation

So, in normal local circulation, plasma proteins are found in high concentrations within the capillaries but in low concentrations in the interstitial space. When injury occurs, swelling results because the damaged capillary wall allows fluid (largely plasma proteins) to leak into the interstitial space.

Meanwhile, the normal inflammatory process begins at the injury site, starting the healing process. Substances released during the inflammatory process that cause pain also cause plasma proteins to leak more readily from the capillaries. Therefore, the damaged capillary wall allows a tremendous amount of fluid to leave the capillaries and fill the interstitial space. The greater the damage, the more fluid that escapes. This fluid in the interstitial space is what you see as acute swelling.

With an understanding of what causes swelling, let's now look at popular methods that you and your athletes' rehabilitation specialists can use to decrease swelling.

HOW COLD MODALITIES DECREASE SWELLING

Physiological effects that help to decrease swelling by the local application of cold are

- decreased circulation,
- decreased inflammation after acute injury, and
- decreased local metabolism.

Decreased Circulation

The application of ice to a body part causes superficial vessels in that area to become narrower, or to constrict, in response to the cold. This process is called *vasoconstriction*. When the diameter of the vessel bringing blood to an area is decreased, less fluid is able to travel through it.

Short-term application of ice is an effective vasoconstrictor. However, some rehabilitation specialists question whether ice should be applied for more than 30 minutes. Early studies demonstrated a reflex increase of circulation due to *vasodilation* (vessels increasing in diameter) following the prolonged application of ice to an area. This response to prolonged cold is termed the *Hunting reflex*. Recently, better controlled studies have refuted the Hunting reflex and show that cold application, even for extended periods, acts as a vasoconstrictor and not a vasodilator.

Decreased Inflammation After Acute Injury

As described in chapter 4, one of the body's natural, local responses to soft-tissue injury is the release of histamine and other substances at the site of injury. These substances are necessary for early healing, but they also bring about local tissue inflammation. If blood flow to an injured area is decreased, fewer of these substances will be released.

Decreased Local Metabolism

Along with decreasing acute inflammation, cold decreases local metabolism. When swelling occurs in response to injury, the increased fluid inhibits adequate circulation to the injured area, and tissue damage results from insufficient oxygen being supplied to the tissue. This process is called *secondary hypoxic injury*. Ice application can circumvent this response by facilitating local healing and thus decreasing the injured tissues' need for oxygen.

Other physiological effects of therapeutic cold that are helpful in the management of athletic injury are

- decreased pain and
- decreased muscle spasm.

Decreased Pain

Ice applied to the skin elicits a predictable sequence of perceived sensations. Initially, the ice is sensed as cold, then as burning and stinging, and finally as a numbing sensation. This numbness results from decreased blood flow to the sensory nerves and an accompanying decrease in the speed (conduction velocity) of the nerve in carrying its pain messages to the brain's sensory cortex. The longer that ice is left on an area, the greater the numbing effect.

Decreased Muscle Spasm

One proposed mechanism to explain how ice decreases spasm is through the decrease of the inflammatory process. Substances released as a result of inflammation cause pain, which as we have seen, causes muscle spasm. Therefore, the application of ice as an anti-inflammatory agent may cause muscle relaxation. Cold also decreases muscle contraction, which is another proposed manner by which ice decreases spasm. Ice also slows nerve conduction, and this too may play a part in decreasing muscle spasm.

PRICE

The exact mechanism by which ice is responsible for decreasing muscle spasm is still being debated. However, ice's ability to decrease inflammation, muscle contractions, and nerve conduction is undoubtedly related to reduced muscle spasm.

COLD MODALITIES

The most frequently used method of delivering therapeutic cold to an injured body part is ice application. Its popularity stems from several factors. I have described how ice helps to decrease swelling by narrowing the vessels carrying fluid to an injured area. And ice is readily available, easy to use, and inexpensive.

Ice is often used by athletes in the form of commercially available cold packs, frozen gel wraps, and ice water whirlpools. However, no matter how cold is applied, the physiological effects are the same.

As with other modalities, ice is only part of the answer. Excessive emphasis should not be placed on only one therapeutic modality to decrease swelling. External compression is another viable option in attempting to control swelling.

Ice Versus Compression

Some researchers and clinicians debate which modality is more beneficial in the management of acute swelling: ice or compression. There is evidence that ice decreases local blood flow and thus swelling. However, it has also been demonstrated that athletes treated with both ice and compression experience less swelling than those treated with ice alone.

Because both modalities should be used routinely and often conjunctively in the management of swelling, let's take a closer look at each modality. Then you'll better understand when cryotherapy, compression, or both should be applied to your injured athletes.

Cryotherapy

Cryotherapy is the general term for the therapeutic use of cold. Protection, rest, compression, and elevation can maximize the effect of cryotherapy in acute injury. The primary effect of ice as a mode of decreasing swelling in acute injury is the subject of this section and, as you read, keep in mind that ice is also used in acute and subacute injury management to decrease pain and muscle spasm.

The most common ways that cold is applied during the rehabilitation process are through

- ice bags,
- ice packs, and
- ice massage.

Ice Bags

The ice bag is probably the simplest and least expensive means of applying cold. Disposable plastic bags of varying sizes to hold the ice are readily available and are inexpensive. The bag should preferably have no leaks. All air should be removed from the bag before sealing or closing it.

Crushed or shaved ice conforms very well to the body part being treated, thereby cooling the area more uniformly. Ice cubes can also be used in disposable plastic bags or commercially available rubber containers that can be easily opened and closed. It is wise when using ice cubes to add a small amount of water to the bag for a more uniform distribution of cold. Ice bags containing ice cubes, crushed or shaved ice, and ice water should be placed directly on the skin over the involved body part.

Although a bit more messy, you may place the ice in a towel if no ice bags are available. The towel should be wetted to facilitate more efficient cooling.

Ice Packs

The ice pack is a self-contained reusable or disposable source of cold. Reusable ice packs contain a gel that can be cooled to low temperatures without becoming frozen solid. This allows the pack to be molded to the shape of the area to be treated. These packs can get very cold, depending on the temperature of the freezer the pack is stored in and the substance frozen. When using this type of cold pack, you should place a damp towel between the skin and the pack to prevent frostbite.

Disposable cold packs are small, self-contained plastic bags that contain ammonia nitrate crystals or beads and a smaller bag of water. Squeezing the smaller bag causes it to burst and then mix with the crystals, thus initiating a chemical reaction that produces a cold liquid.

These packs may also be applied next to the skin; but caution should be used because the liquid produced may cause skin irritation and possibly a chemical burn of the skin exposed directly to the liquid. Although these packs are convenient, their effectiveness is limited in that they often do not maintain cold for a sufficient period of time.

Ice Massage

For small areas, a local ice massage is an alternative mode of cryotherapy. Ice massage may not be recommended in acute injury if the involved body part does not tolerate direct pressure. This is particularly true over bony areas such as the ankle or elbow. However, less bony joints and areas of soft-tissue injury respond well to ice massage.

Here are the steps to take when an ice massage is indicated as part of the injury treatment:

1. Fill a small paper or Styrofoam cup with water to approximately 1 inch from the top of the cup.
2. Place the cup in a freezer until the water is frozen solid.
3. Tear away the top portion of the cup, leaving 1 to 2 inches of ice exposed.
4. Hold the bottom half of the cup and apply the exposed ice to the affected body part by rubbing the ice over the area; the ice will melt quickly until the skin over the area begins to cool.
5. Briskly wipe off the water as it accumulates during the massage to facilitate more efficient cooling.
6. Continue the cycle of massaging and quickly wiping off the water until the treated area becomes numb.

Styrofoam cups seem to work better than paper cups, which tend to stick to the ice. Styrofoam also offers more insulation from the cold to the fingers of the person performing the massage.

Additional Suggestions for Cryotherapy

The injured area should be elevated above the level of the athlete's heart and adequate compression applied. Keep ice on the involved area for 20 to 30 minutes or until the area is numb.

During cold application, the athlete will typically feel this progression of sensations on the area:

1. **Feeling of cold**
2. **Burning and stinging**
3. **Aching**
4. **Numbness**

When icing a joint to decrease swelling, you can remove the ice two or three times during the treatment and have the athlete actively move the joint for a few seconds to allow a more uniform cooling.

After ice treatments, the area treated should be inspected for skin condition. The skin should be reddened (erythematous) over the area to which the ice was applied. You can test this by applying pressure with a fingertip to the reddened area and then removing this pressure. The area previously under the finger should be white. This phenomenon is called *blanching*. After the skin turns white when the pressure is released, it should immediately turn red again.

When the cryotherapy treatment is over, the athletes should rest and elevate the injury until the next treatment, which should begin approximately 2 hours later. After acute injury, however, ice should be used every 1 or 2 hours for the first 48 to 72 hours or until the swelling is gone.

Common Conditions for Cryotherapy

Athletes are most likely to benefit from cryotherapy

- for acute ligament sprains and muscle strains;
- after athletic activity for overuse injuries such as bursitis, tendinitis, sprains, and strains;
- after therapeutic exercise programs for joint and muscle pathology;
- in conjunction with a therapeutic exercise program (cryokinetics); and
- when cold is applied over large superficial blood vessels (groin, armpit, behind the knees) to cool an athlete suffering from heat disorders.

Contraindications for Cryotherapy

General contraindications for cryotherapy include

- cold hypersensitivity,
- Raynaud's disease,
- cardiac disorders, and
- poor circulation.

Cold hypersensitivity. Some individuals are abnormally sensitive to cold. Usually, the hypersensitive reaction results from the release of certain substances that are found naturally in the body but that in this case have an adverse effect on body function. These substances include histamine and other histamine-like chemicals that primarily affect small blood vessels (capillaries) and smooth muscle.

Common symptoms of cold hypersensitivity include redness, itching, a flushed face, sweating, puffy eyelids, abdominal pain, diarrhea, and vomiting. More severe cases may produce shocklike symptoms of decreased blood pressure, increased heart rate, and loss of consciousness. Although cold hypersensitivity is rare, it may be a life-threatening condition, and appropriate medical attention should be sought immediately.

Raynaud's disease. Raynaud's disease is caused by spasm of smooth muscle in the arteries and arterioles of the fingers and toes. Symptoms of numbness, blanching, and pain usually occur in the individual's hands and feet. If an athlete suffers from Raynaud's, cryotherapy should not be used.

Cardiac disorders. Other naturally occurring bodily substances thought to be responsible for cold hypersensitivity may also have a direct effect on blood cells, antibodies, and plasma proteins. The resulting symptoms may include anemia, chills and fever, and heart-rate and blood-pressure changes. These symptoms, as well as the others previously mentioned, may stress the cardiac system excessively when cryotherapy is used on individuals with elevated blood pressure and coronary heart disease.

Poor circulation. Cold should not be used over areas of decreased local circulation or decreased sensation. The inability to adequately sense cold temperature predisposes the athlete to frostbite.

Precautions for Cryotherapy

Care should be taken when using cryotherapy, and extreme caution should be exercised when ice is placed in areas over large superficial nerves. The lateral (outer) area of the knee and the medial (inner) area of the elbow are prime areas of concern. Prolonged (more than a few hours) ice application to these areas has resulted in varying degrees of muscle paralysis and sensory changes.

> Ice should never be applied for more than 20 to 30 minutes, especially over the lateral area of the knee and medial area of the elbow.

To prevent frostbite, a wet towel should be used between the skin and a commercial, refrigerated cold pack.

COMPRESSION

Continuous or intermittent compression is another valuable modality used to decrease swelling. As I described previously, local tissue injury causes fluid to accumulate in the interstitial space. The goal of external compression is to increase pressure of the interstitial fluid, thus forcing the fluid to areas of lower pressure (i.e., lymph vessels, capillaries, and tissue spaces) located away from the injury site. Whether it be constant or intermittent, compression is a vital step in the management of swelling.

Constant Compression

Constant external compression is applied by an outside force to the involved swollen area and kept at a constant pressure. Examples of constant external compression are

- elastic bandages,
- tape, and
- pressure dressings.

Elastic Bandages

Elastic bandages are commonly used to help decrease swelling. The bandage applied to a swollen body part should be of appropriate size. Elastic wraps come in a variety of widths. Table 6.1 lists common bandage widths for various body parts.

Tension in the wrap should be firm but not excessively restricting. If the wrap has been laundered a time or two, much of the elasticity may be lost; these wraps should be discarded. Elastic wraps, like all forms of continuous compression, should be applied after swelling-reducing treatments.

Table 6.1
Widths of Elastic Wrap for Specific Areas

Widths (in.)	Involved body part
3	Foot
	Hand
	Wrist
4	Ankle
	Arm (upper)
	Calf
	Elbow
	Forearm
	Knee (small)
	Shoulder
6	Groin/hip
	Knee (large)
	Thigh

When applying, start at the portion of the involved body part farthest from the heart. Apply firm compression as you wrap the involved area at an angle, or spirally (see Figure 6.1). By applying the wrap this way, fluid is encouraged to move in the proper direction. When the wrap is applied around the swollen body part in a circular rather than a spiral fashion, the bandage tends to produce a tourniquet effect, decreasing its effectiveness (see Figure 6.2).

Tape

Taping techniques can also provide a good form of constant compression. But it is especially important to minimize the potential tourniquet effect of the tape. You can do this by keeping the number of strips of tape that completely encircle the involved body part to a minimum, thus leaving space to which the swelling can migrate (see Figure 6.3). The tourniquet effect is also avoided by using tape

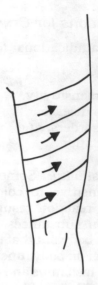

Figure 6.1. Proper alignment of a circumferential compression wrap. Start away from the injury site and apply uniform compression in a spiral manner.

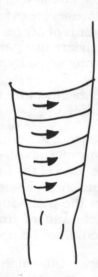

Figure 6.2. Improper alignment of a circumferential compression wrap. Wrapping directly around the injured area in this manner creates circular compression that may inhibit circulation.

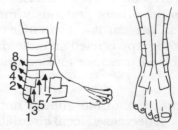

Figure 6.3. Use of tape to provide constant compression. The open basket weave technique used after ankle injury minimizes swelling.

with an elastic component, such as J-Flex (Johnson & Johnson) and Conform (Bike).

Pressure Dressings

Pressure dressings are best utilized underneath elastic wraps, elastic stockinettes, or tape. The ideal pressure dressing conforms to the body part, exerts uniform pressure, and is lightweight. Commercially available products that help satisfy these criteria include orthopedic felt and different types of foam padding of various densities. Some of these materials are even precut for given body parts.

One of the most frequently used pressure-dressing materials is Plastizote. This material is of varying thicknesses and can be heated in a conventional oven to make it pliable. The pliable form is molded to the shape of the body part being treated. When the material cools to room temperature, it retains the form to which it was molded.

A few types of intermittent compression units are available. Although some have different features, all are similar to the one illustrated in Figure 6.4.

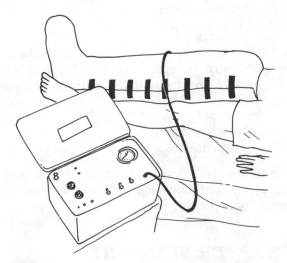

Figure 6.4. Portable intermittent compression unit.

A small, electrically operated portable pump is used to generate the pressure. To this quiet, accurate unit a flexible rubber tube is attached. A sleeve is placed over the body part being treated, to which the opposite end of the rubber tube is attached. The sleeve is an enclosed, inflatable, form-fit air bladder into which the athlete places the involved body part. Air from the pump is forced into the sleeve to a specified pressure, held at that pres-

sure for a pre-set time (usually 10 to 15 seconds), and then released. The treated body part is elevated above the level of the heart and the pressure adjusted to allow for pumping and relaxation.

Intermittent compression is usually kept on the swollen body part 30 to 60 minutes and is often applied in conjunction with cryotherapy. In fact, some intermittent compression units circulate cold liquid through their inflatable sleeves to provide simultaneous cryotherapy.

> To prevent a tourniquet effect, pressures of the intermittent compression unit are not to be set above the athlete's diastolic blood pressure.

HIGH-VOLTAGE GALVANIC STIMULATION

The restoration of normal fluid mechanics is vital in the management of acute injury as well as in other conditions that produce swelling. Compression assists in restoring normal fluid dynamics by applying direct pressure on the swollen area to discourage fluid leakage from the capillary into the interstitial space.

High-voltage galvanic stimulation (HVGS) is also used to help decrease the leakage of fluid into the interstitial space. Whereas compression utilizes mechanical force (pressure) to help restore normal fluid mechanics, HVGS utilizes electrical current to help do the same.

Following are some conditions for which HVGS is commonly used:

- Areas of acute edema caused by ligament sprains or muscle strains
- Soft-tissue overuse injuries such as tendinitis, bursitis, and chronic strains and sprains
- Acute, painful, nonswollen joint pathology
- Muscle reeducation after surgery or prolonged immobilization

How HVGS Decreases Swelling

As discussed earlier, in normal fluid mechanics plasma proteins do not readily pass through capillary pores. These plasma proteins carry a negative electrical charge. Therefore, the environment within capillaries is predominantly negatively charged. After injury, plasma proteins leave the capillaries easily, and the proteins and other substances fill the interstitial space. Because positive charges repel positive charges and negative charges repel negative charges, theoretically a negative charge applied over an injured area should discourage the escape of negatively charged plasma proteins from the capillaries. This is one proposed mechanism whereby HVGS aids in decreasing swelling.

Another postulate as to why HVGS helps decrease swelling is based on studies demonstrating the effects of positive and negative electrical currents on blood clotting. Specific properties of negative and positive charges on fluid dynamics and clotting include those listed below.

The Effects of Electrical Charges on the Body

Positive charge	Negative charge
Facilitates blood clotting	Inhibits blood clotting
Increases tissue stiffness	Decreases tissue stiffness
Attracts acids	Repels acids
Attracts hydrogen ions	Attracts oxygen ions
Repels alkalies	Attracts alkalies

One other theory proposed to explain the effect of HVGS on swelling is that the current from the HVGS may directly stimulate the autonomic nervous system, thus producing vasoconstriction.

Although the exact mechanism by which HVGS decreases swelling is still not fully understood, clinical results are favorable regarding the use of this modality on acute and recurrent swelling.

The HVGS unit is a versatile mode of electrical stimulation. Most units are portable, consistent in application, and easy to use. The HVGS is a unique form of electrical stimulation in that its wave form, pulse width, and pulse rate allow for maximum penetration of soft tissue with minimal discomfort. A wide variety of treatment parameters can be ad-

justed independently of one another; thus, the rehabilitation specialist is afforded many options in treating your athletes with HVGS.

The HVGS current can be applied continuously or can be pulsed so that the current is automatically cycled on and off. The effects of HVGS on swelling are most favorable in the pulsed mode. The desired physiological effect can be obtained by using pulsed current of a net positive or negative charge. Current is applied to the affected body part by electrodes, which are applied directly over the involved area and can be incorporated into an ice-compression wrap or placed inside the inflatable sleeve used with intermittent compression. The HVGS is also commonly used in conjunction with a cold whirlpool and simultaneous active ROM exercises. Treatment times are usually 20 to 30 minutes when applied in conjunction with cryotherapy or can be up to 1 hour when combined with elevation and intermittent compression.

Contraindications and Precautions for HVGS

Although effective in reducing swelling, HVGS should not be applied

- over the heart or the carotid sinus (blood pressure receptors in the front of the neck) or on individuals who have pacemakers,
- over a pregnant uterus,
- across the brain, or
- over a cancerous area.

In addition, HVGS and other forms of electrical therapies should be used with extreme caution in the presence of water.

CHAPTER SUMMARY

1. Swelling is a common condition resulting from sport injury that must be addressed in sport rehabilitation.
2. The two most common methods employed to decrease swelling are cryotherapy (application of cold) and external compression.
3. Local cold can be applied by ice packs, ice bags, ice massage, or ice water immersion.
4. The general effects of the local application of therapeutic cold are decreased

circulation (by means of vasoconstriction), pain, local tissue metabolism, muscle spasm, and acute inflammation.

5. Compression to an injured area to decrease swelling can be constant or intermittent.

6. High-voltage galvanic stimulation (HVGS) is also frequently used alone or in conjunction with compression, cryotherapy, or both.

7. Active muscle movement is the most effective method to circulate fluid within the venous system. Any modalities designed to decrease swelling should be combined with active muscle movement.

Chapter 7

Modalities to Increase Circulation

Circulation, or blood flow, to a given area is increased by a number of different mechanisms, one of which is heat. In this chapter, I examine only the heating of the peripheral (superficial) parts of the body. Peripheral heating differs from changing the body's core, or internal, temperature. Although the measurement of core temperature is vital in assessing some of the medical conditions experienced by athletes, it is beyond the scope of this book.

PRINCIPLES AND ALTERNATIVES IN THERAPEUTIC HEAT APPLICATION

Before I discuss specific modalities to increase circulation, you should know some general principles for applying therapeutic heat to the peripheral system. Among the principles you should consider is whether the heat should be

- general or local and
- superficial or deep.

General Versus Local Heat Application

Application of heat to the body can range from targeting a specific area to treating the entire body. Using moist heat on an arm or leg limits heat exposure to only that body part. Thus, the physiological effects stay local as well. Conversely, when the entire body is immersed in a whirlpool, all body parts are exposed to the heat. Thus, a general effect is realized on the entire body.

Heat should not be used over or on areas of the body that have the following conditions:

- Decreased or absent sensation
- Poor circulation
- Active bleeding
- Recent injury
- Active tumor

In addition, heat should not be applied directly to the abdomen of a pregnant female or to the gonads of a male or female.

Superficial Versus Deep Heat Application

Therapeutic heating effects are usually categorized as superficial or deep. Therefore, in discussing heat as an agent to increase circulation, I identify the heating modalities as either superficial or deep.

Superficial heating refers to the heating of tissue at a depth of 1 centimeter or less. Common modes of superficial heat are hydrocollator packs, paraffin, moist air, fluidotherapy, and hydrotherapy.

Deep heating refers to raising tissue temperature at a depth greater than 1 centimeter. The most frequently used modality for deep heating is ultrasound.

Convection Versus Conduction Versus Conversion Heat Production

The manner in which therapeutic heat is produced must be considered when selecting a modality to increase circulation. Three ways heat may be generated are by

- convection,
- conduction, and
- conversion.

Convection

Convection refers to heating that occurs as a result of heating-medium movement. Heat from the medium (usually air or water) flows to the recipient of the treatment. Convection usually produces a superficial heat. Examples of heating by convection are whirlpools, moist air treatments, and fluidotherapy.

Conduction

Heat is transferred by *conduction* when there is an actual exchange of energy within an object or from one object to another object in close proximity. This energy exchange occurs as high energy molecules pass to lower energy molecules (energy from a hot area to a colder area). Examples of heating by conduction are hot packs, hot water bottles, and paraffin baths. Heating by conduction usually results in increased superficial circulation.

Conversion

Conversion occurs when one form of energy is converted into another form of energy. Common modes of conversion heating occur as nonthermal energy (electrical, mechanical, or electromagnetic) is converted into thermal energy. The most common example of heating by conversion is ultrasound. Heating by conversion typically promotes deep circulation.

THE EFFECTS OF THERAPEUTIC HEAT

Although the mechanics involved in the production of heat vary, the general desired physiological effects of therapeutic heat are similar and include the following:

- Enhanced stretching ability of tissues

- Decreased pain
- Decreased muscle spasm
- Decreased inflammation
- Increased blood flow
- Relaxation

Enhanced Stretching Ability of Tissues

Researchers have speculated that heat makes the nerves that are responsible for muscle activity less likely to signal the muscle to contract, thereby decreasing muscle tone. And, without a doubt, heat helps increase the ability of tissue to be stretched. Thus, heating is a desirable component of a successful stretching program.

Decreased Pain

Heat can decrease pain directly by its effect on nerve conduction. Heat decreases the sensitivity of fast-twitch nerve fibers, which are responsible for sensing touch. Prolonged application of heat also decreases the sensitivity of slow-twitch fibers and thereby inhibits pain messages to the brain.

Decreased Muscle Spasm

As noted in chapter 4, ischemia and muscle spasm are highly interrelated. Heat, as a vasodilator, brings more blood to an area and thus serves to decrease local tissue ischemia. Therefore, an increase in circulation and a subsequent decrease in ischemia yields decreased muscle spasm.

Decreased Inflammation

After injury to soft tissue, the tissue structures bleed from the site of damage to local blood vessels. To stop the blood flow, the body's intricate clotting mechanism is activated, and damaged cells from the area combine with blood cells to form a blood clot. Substances from the damaged cells are subsequently released and cause an inflammatory response in the area of injury. Other enzymes are released to assist the healing process and stimulate the nerves responsible for sending pain sensations to the brain.

This natural inflammatory response can be minimized by the use of heat. Increased local blood flow stimulated by the application of heat helps the body resolve these substances by bringing in blood to wash away the agents responsible for pain, swelling, and inflammation. Thus, heat may serve as an anti-inflammatory agent.

However, using heat too soon will actually slow down the body's attempt to start the healing process. Applying heat to an injured site before adequate clotting has begun causes clotting to be retarded. Excess fluid is then allowed to enter the interstitial space, resulting in swelling.

Increased Blood Flow

Perhaps the most popular rationale for using heat is the effect on the spasm and ischemia components of the pain-spasm-ischemia cycle. By causing the blood vessels in the injured area to dilate, more blood flows to the immediate area, thus helping to counteract the local tissue ischemia that results from injury.

Relaxation

The soothing effect of heat on muscle spasm, pain, and nerve sensitivity produces an overall effect of relaxation.

TYPES OF HEAT MODALITIES

Heat-generating modalities may affect injured tissues superficially or deeply. The modality needed for your injured athletes depends on the type, severity, and phase of the injury. So let's examine the various modes of superficial and deep heating, and you'll better understand which modality is appropriate for your next injury situation.

Superficial Heating Modalities

Now that you have an idea of the general categories of heat, how heat may be transferred, and the effects of heat, let's look at a few superficial heating modalities commonly

used in the management of athletic injury. Although these methods are frequently applied by the sports medicine specialist, you should be familiar with them as well. Superficial heating methods not discussed in this section but available to your athletes include moist heating pads, hot towels, and a good old-fashioned hot bath.

Hydrocollator Packs (Hot Packs)

The hot pack is probably the most easily and frequently used source of therapeutic superficial heat. A hot pack is a canvas structure of varying dimensions (standard size is 9 by 9 inches) and shapes that allows for the treatment of any body part. The packs are constructed of individual compartments, each 1-1/2 inches wide and containing a silica-based compound that, when immersed in water, becomes gellike. The packs are kept in a self-contained, electrically operated unit called a *hydrocollator*. Water temperature is thermostatically controlled at approximately 165 °F. The silica gel allows the pack to hold the hot water and retain its heat for 15 to 20 minutes.

Six to eight layers of toweling should be placed between the injured body part and the hot pack. Custom-made, commercially available hot pack covers of heavy toweling are often used to accommodate the different hot pack shapes.

Hot packs relax superficial muscles and increase superficial blood flow, as evidenced by the erythema (redness) of the tissue it is applied to. Hot packs should be applied to an area for 20 minutes every 4 hours. Prolonged (longer than 20 minutes) or more frequent (within 4 hours) application of hot packs does not affect the depth of heat penetration (about 1 centimeter maximum), and maximum skin temperature is attained after approximately 8 minutes. Thus prudent and timely use of hot packs will achieve the same benefits as extensive, repeated applications.

Hot packs also decrease the electrical resistance of the skin and thus are commonly used before ultrasound.

Because of their ease of application and inexpensive cost, hot packs are very useful in the management of many sport injuries.

The use of hydrocollator packs is especially beneficial in the following conditions:

- Superficial muscle spasm, strain, and tendinitis

- In conjunction with ultrasound for deep-muscle spasm, strain, and tendinitis
- Delayed muscle soreness
- Before stretching

Paraffin

Paraffin baths are small, self-contained units but are usually large enough to immerse the lower arm, the foot, or the ankle. Some units are smaller and allow only the hand and wrist to be treated.

These units are thermostatically controlled to heat a mixture of paraffin wax and mineral oil to approximately 126 °F. The affected body part is then dipped into the hot liquid mixture and is either removed immediately or kept there for 15 to 20 minutes. The part is removed for only 3 to 5 seconds, which is sufficient time for the liquid to harden and another waxy layer to be added. Repetitive dips, usually 10 to 15, are performed until a thick coating is created. The affected part is then wrapped in layers of toweling, usually for 15 to 20 minutes, to help retain the heat. When the treatment is complete, the paraffin slides off the body like a glove.

Considering paraffin's low heat-carrying capacity, you might think that the potential benefit of this modality as a heat source is limited. However, this modality raises tissue temperature very effectively. The temperature of the paraffin is 126 °F, but, because of the substance's low heat conductivity, this high temperature is tolerated well. Skin exposed to water at 126 °F, however, will not tolerate the treatment because of water's higher specific heat and heat conductivity. Therefore, when a higher temperature is desired in the skin, paraffin is a wise choice.

Contraindications for paraffin use are similar to those for general therapeutic heating. *Open wounds should not be treated with paraffin baths.*

Paraffin is commonly used for the following conditions:

- After prolonged immobilization of a wrist or hand
- As an adjunct to joint mobilization and stretching of the wrist and hand
- For tendinitis of the wrist, hand, ankle, and toes

Hydrotherapy (Warm or Hot Whirlpool)

The whirlpool treatments discussed in this section include only warm and hot water hydrotherapies (temperatures from 93 °F to 106 °F). Cool and cold water whirlpools were discussed in the previous chapter.

Whirlpools are available in all shapes and sizes. Extremity tanks, which allow a lower leg or an entire arm to be treated, are commonly used in the treatment of athletes. A low-boy whirlpool is similar to a bathtub and allows at least the lower half of the body to be completely immersed. Some whirlpools are large enough to allow walking in chest-deep water. Hubbard tanks allow for total body immersion with enough room for simultaneous full (arm and leg) ROM exercises.

Most whirlpools can be adjusted to allow air to be mixed into the water and to vary the force of water exiting the agitator. The greater the amount of air and the force of water exiting the agitator, the greater the mechanical effect of the water on the skin.

Superficial heating modalities are designed to heat the body's periphery. However, immersing large body areas in a hot or warm whirlpool may affect the body's core temperature. The greater the temperature of the water and the greater the body area immersed, the greater the increase in core temperature.

Water temperature guidelines for whirlpool treatments include the following:

- When immersing a single body part (e.g., a foot and an ankle or a hand and a wrist), the temperature of the water may range from 104 °F to 106 °F.
- When the entire arm or the leg from the thigh down is underwater, the temperature should be between 102 °F and 104 °F.
- When the entire body is being immersed, whirlpool temperatures should not exceed 100 °F.
- Normal treatment time at all temperatures should range from 20 to 30 minutes.

Note: Some researchers have suggested higher temperatures—up to

115 °F for a single limb and 105 °F for a total body treatment. In a healthy athlete these higher temperatures may be well tolerated and used with caution.

In addition to providing relaxation and increasing superficial circulation, whirlpools may be used in the management of open wounds. Water temperature during open-wound treatment should be between 96 °F and 98 °F. More important, care must be taken to keep the whirlpool clean. The whirlpool should be sterilized by running a cleaning solution through the agitator. An antiseptic solution should also be added to the water during the treatment. Also, after open wound treatment, the whirlpool should be scrubbed manually to ensure that the inside of the tank is clean.

General precautions regarding heat apply also to the whirlpool. However, a few additional precautions need to be kept in mind:

- Keep the whirlpool clean.
- Make sure the whirlpool's electrical system is grounded safely.
- Keep all electrical appliances away from the whirlpool area.
- Never leave an athlete alone in a whirlpool.
- Make sure all temperature-monitoring equipment functions properly.
- Do not exceed temperature or time guidelines.

The whirlpool can be a handy source of heat, relaxation, and healing for the following conditions:

- Sprains and strains that are at least 48 to 72 hours old
- After prolonged immobilization
- After surgery (stitches should be out and wounds closed)
- Skin lacerations, scrapes, cuts, and blisters
- Before stretching
- Painful or weak extremities that have limited ROM

Deep-Heating Modalities

Many tissues injured in athletic events are located deeper than 1 centimeter. As we have seen, superficial heat may effectively prepare an area for deep heat but is able to penetrate only about 1 centimeter. Thus, deep-heating modalities are required to deliver heat to tissues below 1 centimeter.

Because these treatment modalities penetrate to greater depths, there is a greater risk of potential injury to the athlete if the modalities are misused. Therefore, the use of deep-heating modalities is restricted to trained sports medicine specialists.

Ultrasound

Although you should not perform ultrasound treatments on your athletes, ultrasound is the most frequently used source of deep heat in sport rehabilitation. Ultrasound, as a source of therapeutic heat, produces good results when used appropriately. And, because your athletes may need such treatment, a brief introduction is in order.

The ultrasound unit is lightweight and portable and houses the mechanics to generate an adjustable source of sound waves. Attached to the unit is the sound head, or transducer, which delivers the heat (energy) to the involved body part. The unit produces high-frequency sound waves of approximately 1 megacycle (1 million cycles per second). These sound waves penetrate the skin and reach the layer of tissue below. Different body tissues, such as skin, fat, fascia, muscle, and bone, have different densities. As the sound waves penetrate a tissue layer of one density, some of the waves continue into the next layer; however, some of them are unable to penetrate and are reflected back. This reflection of waves between two layers of tissue of different densities produces heat. Therefore, ultrasound creates deep heat by converting mechanical energy (sound waves) to heat.

A coupling medium (commercially available gels or mineral oil) is required for ultrasound to be transmitted from the sound head to the body part.

Treatments of areas with irregular contours are done underwater. In this case, the sound head is held approximately 1 inch away from the injured body part, and the water serves as the coupling medium.

Because therapeutic doses of heat produced by ultrasound often penetrate up to 5 centimeters and can elevate temperatures 2 °F to

3 °F, ultrasound is a very potent and efficient source of deep heat. Depending on the treatment needed, pulsed or continuous ultrasound may be used.

Pulsed ultrasound yields less of a temperature buildup and therefore can be used for a longer treatment period. Also, because less heat builds up, pulsed sound may be used earlier in the injury management process than continuous ultrasound.

Continuous ultrasound has a more pronounced heating effect than pulsed sound, and treatment times are generally shorter. An area approximately the size of a fist should be treated continuously for no more than 5 minutes.

Ultrasound can produce the following physiological effects:

- An increase in the level of cortisol, a potent, naturally occurring anti-inflammatory agent
- An elevated temperature in a joint capsule located deep in the body (hip or shoulder) and in deep scar tissue
- A decrease in tissue oxygen consumption
- An increased ability of tissue to be penetrated (an important function discussed under the topic of phonophoresis in chapter 8)

As with superficial heating modalities, ultrasound should not be used on recently injured tissue, body areas with diminished sensation, a developing fetus, an active tumor, or the gonads. Additional contraindications include the following:

- Ultrasound should not be used over the eyes.
- Care should be used when treating over the growth plates of maturing bones.
- Ultrasound should be used with caution around the heart, the endocrine glands (kidney and neck regions), and the central nervous system.

Ultrasound is an effective modality for treating the following conditions:

- Joint contractures and inflammation
- Bursitis
- Nerve inflammation
- Deep-muscle strains, tendinitis, contractures, resolved contusions, and myofascial pain
- Muscle spasm
- Subacute and chronic ligament sprains
- Plantar warts
- Stiffness before therapeutic exercise to stretch or strengthen

CHAPTER SUMMARY

1. Heating modalities increase circulation by means of vasodilation. An increase in circulation can be local (concentrated on a given body part) or generalized (having an effect on the entire body by affecting core temperature).
2. Therapeutic heat can be classified as superficial or deep. Superficial heating refers to elevating tissue temperature at a depth of 1 centimeter or less, whereas deep heating refers to heating tissue at a depth greater than 1 centimeter.
3. Therapeutic heat can be transferred to the body by convection, conduction, or conversion.
4. Therapeutic heat serves to decrease pain, muscle spasm, and inflammation by increasing blood flow. Increased blood flow enhances the ability of tissue to be stretched and promotes general relaxation.
5. Superficial heating modalities commonly used in the care of the injured athlete are hydrocollator packs, paraffin, and hydrotherapy.
6. The most common deep-heating modality used in treating injured athletes is ultrasound.

Chapter 8
Modalities to Decrease Pain and Inflammation

Modalities that address the spasm and ischemia components of the pain-spasm-ischemia cycle were discussed in chapters 6 and 7. The primary goal of the treatment modalities discussed to this point has been to increase or decrease temperatures at the injury site. However, the secondary effect of these modalities is to decrease pain.

For example, an athlete who strains a calf muscle may prevent swelling and secondary hypoxic injury by immediately applying an ice bag. Cold also will temporarily slow down the transmission of signals carried by pain nerve fibers, causing decreased pain sensation. Similarly, after the acute phase, moist heat and ultrasound may be used to decrease muscle spasm and facilitate stretching, thereby decreasing discomfort.

THE EXPERIENCE AND RELIEF OF PAIN

Pain is recognized by the brain through a complex series of physiological events. I will try to describe this complicated sequence as simply as possible. A painful stimulus is recognized at the local site of pain by specialized pain receptors called *nociceptors*. These dull, burning, and aching pain sensations then travel by way of peripheral nerves into the spinal column and finally to the sensory cortex of the brain. The peripheral nerve fibers that transmit dull, aching sensations are called C nerve fibers, whereas the nerve fibers that transmit sharp, prickly pain sensations to the spinal column and the brain are called A nerve fibers.

Both dull and sharp pain sensations can be decreased by therapeutic means such as cold, electrical stimulation, and medication. Each of these modalities reduces the irritability of these nerve-carrying pain sensations by altering the body's perception of pain.

MODALITIES TO DECREASE PAIN

A few modalities used in athletic rehabilitation primarily serve to decrease pain. That is, the physiological effect of these modalities is to alter the pain sensation realized by the brain. In turn, pain reduction has a direct effect on muscle relaxation and local circulation. The modalities used in athletic rehabilitation to decrease pain are

- pain medications,
- cryotherapy,
- transcutaneous electrical nerve stimulation, and
- electroacupuncture.

Pain Medications

Pain medications block certain postinjury reactions that result in the perception of pain. Aspirin and other aspirinlike drugs may help relieve pain. These over-the-counter drugs should be used with discretion and only when not contraindicated. Medications more potent than aspirin must not be used without a prescription from a medical doctor. And such drugs should be used only after consulting the prescribing physician.

Cryotherapy

As mentioned previously, ice has an anesthetic effect and thus is an effective modality for decreasing pain. As discussed in chapter 6, ice can be applied by ice packs, ice bags, or ice massage. Two additional methods of cryotherapy are ice water immersion and topical application of cold spray.

Ice Water Immersion

Ice water immersion was purposely not mentioned when discussing cryotherapy modes to decrease swelling because, although this method is frequently used for generalized muscle soreness at cool rather than cold temperatures, it is not recommended for acute injury. This is because the foot, ankle, elbow, wrist, or hand, when being treated, is placed in a dependent position, in which the body part to be treated is below the level of the heart. Even when a healthy (noninjured) body part is left in a dependent position, the efficiency of venous and lymphatic return is decreased because of gravity. Therefore, when a body part is swollen, the return of fluid into the circulatory system is further compromised.

Contrast Bath

A variation of ice water immersion is the contrast bath, in which cold and hot water immersion are alternated. But, because the arm or leg is again placed in a dependent position and a modality that increases circulation (hot water) added, contrast baths are rarely prescribed for pain reduction, even during the subacute phase.

As alternatives, ice, constant compression, and elevation work well; intermittent compression and HVGS may provide additional relief. And, when an immediate reduction of pain is the goal, ice bags, ice packs, and ice massages are more convenient and effective than ice water immersion.

Topical Cold Spray Application

When an immediate decrease in discomfort is the goal, topical cold application is a useful modality. Substances commonly used are fluoromethane and ethyl chloride. These substances are in a liquid or an aerosol form; both can be sprayed directly onto the injured body part. Concerns of damage to the atmosphere's ozone layer have helped make fluoromethane the more popular option. This modality can also be costly, so you should be selective in using it.

You should also exercise caution for medical reasons. Contusions to areas covering bony prominences such as the malleolus (ankle), olecranon (elbow), and digits (fingers and toes) are effectively treated with cold spray. The part to be treated is sprayed until numb. However, before you apply the spray, you must be certain that the bony involvement is limited to contusions and is not severe.

> Under no circumstances should cryotherapy be used to numb a painful, unstable joint injury or a significant muscle or tendon problem to allow an athlete to return to competition.

Transcutaneous Electrical Nerve Stimulation (TENS)

Next to ice application, perhaps the second most frequently used therapeutic modality to directly decrease pain is *transcutaneous electrical nerve stimulation* (TENS). This relatively new treatment modality had its real beginnings in the late 1960s. Tremendous progress has made the TENS unit more versatile, lightweight, and sophisticated. Clinically, these units have proven beneficial in managing acute, chronic, and postoperative pain.

A TENS unit is a portable, lightweight, battery-operated apparatus about the size of a pocket pager. The unit is usually clipped to a belt or the waistband of a pair of slacks. Small wires (leads) connect the unit to electrodes that are placed on the athlete's skin. These electrodes, usually about 1-1/4 inches square, are placed over the body part to be stimulated. A low-intensity electrical current is generated by the unit and passes through the athlete's skin by means of the electrodes, hence the name *transcutaneous*. The TENS unit allows current intensity and current pulse width and rate to be adjusted independently.

The TENS unit is utilized while the athlete is experiencing pain. During acute episodes of pain, the unit may be employed continuously over the course of 2 to 3 days until pain has subsided. In cases where motion does not aggravate the injury, the athlete may benefit from active exercises while the TENS unit is applied. However, pain is a warning that lets one know when activity has become too strenuous. Therefore, if the athlete is experiencing pain, no motion exercises should be performed while the TENS unit is operating.

Also, TENS can be a wise alternative to pain medication because it does not have the potential side effects of medications such as drowsiness, lethargy, confusion, and nausea. And, because the unit is portable, the athlete may wear the unit and use it when pain is present and then simply turn it off when pain subsides. In this manner, the athlete can effectively manage his or her pain.

Theoretical Basis of Pain Relief Through TENS

Two prevalent explanations for how TENS decreases pain are the gate control theory and the endogenous opiate theory.

Gate control theory. The C nerve fibers carry the pain sensations experienced in athletic injuries. These fibers are less than 1 micrometer in diameter and lack a special insulation called *myelin*, which allows for the quick conduction of nerve transmission. These C fibers carry their messages to the brain slower than the larger A fibers (1 to 6 micrometers), which are myelinated. Through the stimulation of A fibers with the TENS unit's high-pulse-rate electrical current, messages on the A fibers reach the brain quicker than they do on the C fibers. For example, picture a door or a gate in the brain where sensation is realized. When A fibers are stimulated, this gate in the brain locks in comfortable, tingling sensations and locks out messages of dull, aching pain (traveling on the C fibers). The gate is actually a sophisticated biochemical reaction (the manner in which the nerves respond and pass their information along is beyond the scope of our discussion). Suffice it to say that pain sensation is modulated and clinically decreased by stimulation of the larger fibers by means of the TENS unit.

Endogenous opiate theory. The second mechanism proposed for the decrease of pain through TENS is based on the endogenous opiate theory. Certain substances that are routinely found within the body (endogenous) have a direct pain-reducing effect. These substances are derivatives of chemicals collectively termed *opiates*. Some opiates are similar to the chemical compound morphine but are hundreds of times more potent; these are called *endorphins*. The stimulation of C fibers by low frequencies (less than 4 pulses per second) causes a release of endorphins into the bloodstream. Not surprisingly then, circulatory endorphins have been shown to decrease pain.

In summary, gate control theory holds that A nerve fibers are stimulated with high pulse rates and wide pulse widths, the perceived muscle sensation being a tingle. Endogenous opiate theory holds that C nerve fibers are stimulated with low pulse rates and narrow pulse widths, the perceived muscle sensation being a contraction.

Common uses of TENS include the following:

- Acute or chronic ligament sprain and muscle strain
- Acute contusion of soft tissue
- Peripheral nerve inflammation or radiating pain (radiculopathy)
- Chronic pain and myofascial pain syndrome
- Postoperative incisional pain (immediately after surgery)

Like other forms of electrical stimulation, TENS has precautions and contraindications governing its use. Please refer to those listed under high-voltage galvanic stimulation on page 48.

Electroacupuncture

Another pain-reducing modality that utilizes electrical current is electroacupuncture. An example of this modality is the Neuroprobe. This unit can be operated by battery or off a 110-volt outlet. The tabletop unit is lightweight and portable but is not worn by the athlete as is a TENS unit. The primary use of electroacupuncture is to decrease pain by controlling C-fiber stimulation.

A low-frequency current (less than 4 pulses per second) can be applied using a hand-held stimulator. The current, which stimulates C fibers, is increased until discomfort is felt by the athlete. Maximal endorphins are released by means of the low-frequency stimulus, which is also a noxious stimulus that causes optimal C-fiber response. Local points of discomfort are stimulated, as are acupuncture points and auriculotherapy points, which are sites on the athlete's ear corresponding to the involved area of the body. Generally, acupuncture points are stimulated for 1 minute, and as a rule local points are stimulated for 30 seconds.

Precautions, contraindications, and common conditions treated are similar to those for TENS with the exception of postoperative incisional pain. Electroacupuncture and TENS are not absolutely necessary in the treatment of athletic injury, but they do—when used correctly—treat acute and chronic pain effectively.

MODALITIES TO DECREASE INFLAMMATION

Pain often accompanies acute or chronic inflammation. Acute inflammation is the body's natural reaction to injury at the cellular level. Inflammation results from local cell damage and further insult from secondary hypoxia. Many substances in the body are released at various stages of the inflammatory process. Pain, swelling, loss of function, redness, and warmth of the involved areas are common signs of inflammation.

Oral anti-inflammatory medication is commonly used to decrease inflammation. In addition to superficial and deep heat, other modalities routinely used include phonophoresis, iontophoresis, and microamperage electrical nerve stimulation.

Phonophoresis

Phonophoresis is the use of ultrasound to drive medication through skin and subcutaneous tissues to areas of inflammation or pain. Common anti-inflammatory medications used in phonophoresis are aspirin and hydrocorti-

sone. The medication is usually premixed into a topical cream and then applied to the athlete's skin over the area to be treated. An ultrasound treatment is then performed over the involved area to drive the medication through the skin to deeper layers.

The area to be treated is often heated before phonophoresis is performed for subacute and chronic conditions. Cold packs and phonophoresis are used together in some cases of acute injury. The length of treatment time varies depending on the area being treated but is generally similar to that of traditional ultrasound. Athletes may have allergic reactions to phonophoresis as indicated by red, raised areas that itch. In these cases treatment should not be continued.

General contraindications for the use of ultrasound apply also to phonophoresis. Care must be taken to ensure that the athlete is not allergic to the anti-inflammatory agent. The depth of penetration has been reported to be 5 centimeters, so the long-term use of steroids (e.g., hydrocortisone) warrants special consideration. Many cases of acute tendon rupture have been reported after steroid injection into and around a tendon. Although doses of hydrocortisone delivered to an area by means of phonophoresis are significantly less than those delivered by injection, it is uncertain to what extent tendons are subsequently weakened. Therefore, vigorous eccentric muscle activity may need to be curtailed in these cases.

Other agents that decrease pain are sometimes used with phonophoresis (e.g., lidocaine). In these cases (and with any modality used to numb an area), stresses placed on the area during periods of analgesia or anesthesia should be appropriate. Also, because these substances are medications, treatments must be prescribed by a physician. Especially in the practice of testing athletes for performance-enhancing drugs, the physician will know which drugs and the dosages to use.

Phonophoresis is often utilized for the following conditions:

- Acute and subacute muscle or tendon strain
- Subacute and chronic tendinitis
- Bursitis
- Inflamed plica (synovial thickening of the knee)

- Tenosynovitis (inflamed tendon sheath surrounding a tendon)

Iontophoresis

Iontophoresis is the use of a direct current to drive ions of a particular substance through the skin, subcutaneous tissue, and underlying tissues to a depth of approximately 1 centimeter. The wave form of the direct current provides a net positive or negative charge under a specific electrode. A portable electric stimulator delivers the direct current to the involved area by means of leads and attached electrodes.

Positive charges at the positive electrode that repel like positive ions tend to harden tissue at the area of stimulation and increase nerve irritability. Negative charges at the negative electrode have the opposite effects. The sport rehabilitation specialist applies a positive or negative electrode, depending on the ion to be driven into the affected area. The electrode is placed on the area to be treated. A small, direct current of 5 milliamps or less is then generated by the stimulator, forcing the ions into the skin and subcutaneous tissue.

Common substances used in iontophoresis include

- acetic acid,
- dexamethasone,
- sodium salicylate, and
- xylocaine.

The substance used is usually applied as a weak solution to a gauze pad that is then placed on the skin over the area to be treated. The electrode supplying the desired positive or negative charge is placed over the gauze at the treatment site. Treatment time is usually 15 to 20 minutes. The Phoresor, a special unit to deliver current for iontophoresis is also used. This system is convenient and less cumbersome, but a minimal number of parameters may be adjusted, thus lessening the overall capability of the unit.

Precautions and contraindications of iontophoresis are similar to those of phonophoresis. Careful attention must be paid to the treatment protocol to safeguard against excessive skin irritation and possible burning.

Iontophoresis is used for the same conditions for which phonophoresis is used (see page 60).

Microamperage Electrical Nerve Stimulation (MENS)

Although *microamperage electrical nerve stimulation* (MENS) is not technically an anti-inflammatory modality, a secondary response to this relatively new and effective treatment is the reduction of injury-site inflammation. By enhancing protein synthesis in the treated area, MENS facilitates healing at the cellular level. As healing is facilitated, inflammatory responses are decreased.

Whereas most electrical stimulation units produce milliamperage current, MENS utilizes microamperage current. The current is delivered to the athlete from the MENS unit through leads attached to electrodes that are either attached to the patient or hand held. The hand-held applicators are very versatile in their ability to treat local areas of involvement.

This modality has shown favorable clinical results in treating a variety of acute and chronic conditions. Also, MENS seems to be better tolerated by athletes and to produce better results than milliamperage units.

Popular MENS units are the Mens-O-Matic and the Electro-Acuscope. Precautions, contraindications, and conditions to which MENS therapy applies are similar to those of HVGS, ultrasound, TENS, and phonophoresis.

CONCLUSION

I hope this chapter increased your understanding of the therapeutic modalities available to decrease the pain or inflammation your athletes may experience. It is important that these modalities are recommended and in some cases applied by a sports medicine specialist. It is also critical that the appropriate modality is applied at the proper time during the rehabilitation phase.

For a brief summary of the modalities used during a given phase of a sport rehabilitation program, refer to Table 8.1.

Table 8.1
Modalities Used in Sport Rehabilitation

	Acute phase				Subacute phase				Chronic phase			
	I	P	Sp	Sw	I	P	Sp	Sw	I	P	Sp	Sw
Cold spray	✔	✔										
Diathermy					✔	✔	✔		✔	✔	✔	
Hot packs					✔	✔	✔		✔	✔	✔	
HVGS	✔	✔	✔	✔	✔	✔	✔	✔	✔	✔	✔	✔
Hydrotherapy	✔	✔	✔	✔	✔	✔	✔	✔	✔	✔	✔	✔
Ice packs	✔	✔	✔	✔	✔	✔	✔	✔	✔	✔	✔	✔
Ice massage	✔	✔	✔	✔	✔	✔	✔	✔	✔	✔	✔	✔
Intermittent compression				✔				✔				✔
Iontophoresis	✔	✔			✔	✔			✔	✔		
MENS	✔	✔	✔	✔	✔	✔	✔	✔	✔	✔	✔	✔
Phonophresis		✔			✔	✔	✔		✔	✔	✔	
TENS	✔	✔					✔			✔		
Ultrasound					✔	✔	✔	✔	✔	✔	✔	✔

Note. I = inflammation, P = pain, Sp = spasm, and Sw = swelling.

CHAPTER SUMMARY

1. Therapeutic modalities utilized by the sports medicine specialist are primarily designed to decrease spasm and ischemia. However, two modalities are most frequently applied to decrease pain: transcutaneous electrical nerve stimulation (TENS) and electroacupuncture.
2. Although used primarily to decrease swelling, cryotherapy is another modality used to decrease pain.
3. Pain is one symptom of inflammation. Modalities used to decrease postinjury inflammation are ice and anti-inflammatory agents driven into the skin by ultrasound (phonophoresis) and electrical current (iontophoresis).
4. A new and promising modality designed to facilitate healing and decrease pain and inflammation is microamperage electrical nerve stimulation (MENS).

Part Summary

The judicious use of physical modalities plays an important role in athletic rehabilitation. From playing absolutely vital roles in acute injury management to being small but integral adjuncts in comprehensive sport rehabilitation, therapeutic modalities provide the injured athlete total rehabilitative care. You should evaluate the roles these modalities play at various points in the rehabilitation process to help ensure that your athletes receive appropriate treatment from all the available injury-care technologies.

PART IV

Therapeutic Process of Sport Rehabilitation

Too often in my practice of sport rehabilitation I have seen reinjury result from inadequate rehabilitation. The problem usually is not an improper choice of therapeutic modality or the failure to apply a special brace or support but rather the failure to address the basics of adequate range of motion, muscle strength, and functional ability.

Every sport stresses a given body part in a unique way. Thus, it is not surprising that specific physical problems result from participation in one sport but not another. And, logically, sport-specific injury must be addressed specifically. But far too often, range of motion, strength, and functional evaluations are not based on the specific mechanism of injury and the demands of the sport.

In this part, I share with you the basics of therapeutic exercise in relation to problems frequently encountered in sport rehabilitation. Chapters are devoted to range of motion (flexibility), strength, and joint sense (proprioception).

In the section on range of motion, general guidelines regarding normal flexibility, principles of proper stretching, and methods to improve motion following both acute and chronic injury are described. Common sport injuries that result in decreased range of motion and common conditions in which decreased range of motion contributes to injury are also presented.

The section on strengthening examines muscle contraction relative to the rehabilitation process, strength exercise progression, muscle strength grades, and muscle balance. Common acute and chronic injuries resulting in a loss of muscle strength or muscle balance are discussed, as are approaches for strengthening and restoring balance.

Joint sense, or proprioception, is vital yet often neglected in sport rehabilitation. Special programs to restore joint sense in the upper and lower extremities are addressed in the section regarding this important aspect of the therapeutic process.

As you will see, after range of motion, strength, and proprioception are restored, one more step is required before an athlete is allowed to return to full participation. This stage of the process, called functional progression, involves restoring sport-specific function. But before we examine that final step of sport rehabilitation, you must grasp the elements of a sound therapeutic exercise program.

Chapter 9
Exercises to Increase Range of Motion

Few of us are as limber as we could be; and, through proper exercise, almost everyone could improve the range of motion in their joints. Injured athletes must be particularly concerned about maximizing their range of motion because restricted movement at the injury site can lead to reinjury or, at least, to substandard performance. So take a close look at the following section on range of motion. I am sure you don't want your athletes to be injured or to perform poorly when you could have prevented it.

DEFINING RANGE OF MOTION

For our discussion, *range of motion* (ROM) can be defined as the movement of a body part through a particular joint's complete, unrestricted, normal motion. Normal joint movement is dictated by the following:

- The type of joint involved
- The shape and surface of the joint involved
- The degrees of freedom of motion allowed at the particular joint
- The contractile and noncontractile tissues surrounding the joint

Although a complete description of these factors is beyond the scope of this book, you should understand the basics of joint mechanics presented in this chapter.

TYPES OF RANGE OF MOTION

Normal ROM occurs smoothly when active muscle contraction produces muscle shortening. As the muscle shortens, the bone on which the particular muscle inserts is acted on, yielding physiological joint motion. Normal ROMs have been established for each joint of the body. In discussing the problems frequently encountered by athletes experiencing restricted ROM, I also present the normal ROMs.

Range of motion is categorized as being active, active-assisted, or passive. Active and passive components can be subdivided into physiological and accessory components.

Active Range of Motion

Active range of motion (AROM) is the motion produced by active muscle contraction. Forces generated by the muscle that are primarily responsible for a given motion cause the body segment to which the muscle is inserted to move toward the muscle's origin. Active ROM can occur with the assistance of gravity, with the effect of gravity eliminated, or against gravity. Active ROM must be assessed as the body part moves against gravity, and it provides a true measurement of the muscle and tendon tissue's effect on joint movement.

Active-Assisted Range of Motion

Active-assisted range of motion (AAROM) is motion in which the body segment being moved is assisted through at least part of the normal ROM. Motion must be assisted because of a breakdown in normal ROM. Assistance can be offered by gravity, an uninvolved body part, an object or device, or an external force (see Figure 9.1).

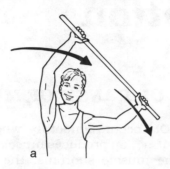

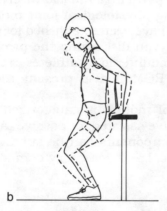

Figure 9.1. Active-assisted ROM: a, using a cane to assist right-shoulder abduction; b, using body weight to assist left-shoulder extension.

Passive Range of Motion

Passive range of motion (PROM) is movement that takes place with no active muscle assistance. It is usually performed by another person who takes the body part through the ROM manually. The athlete may also perform PROM manually on him- or herself.

Physiological and Accessory Motion

Active and passive ROM can be subdivided into *physiological motion* and *accessory motion*. Physiological motions are those that one can perform oneself; they are voluntary. These motions occur in one of the three primary planes of motion—sagittal, transverse, or coronal—or in any combination of these planes (see Figure 9.2).

An example of physiological motion is flexion of the shoulder, which occurs in the sagittal plane (see Figure 9.3). Physiological motions can be performed actively by the athlete, or they may be performed passively as the athlete allows the body part to be moved through a given plane or planes.

Accessory motions differ from physiological motions in that they are automatic and involuntary. These automatic motions take place at the same time that voluntary, physiological motions do. Accessory motions are the gliding, spinning, and rolling components of normal joint motion and are dictated mainly by the shape of the bones that meet at the involved joint. Without accessory motion,

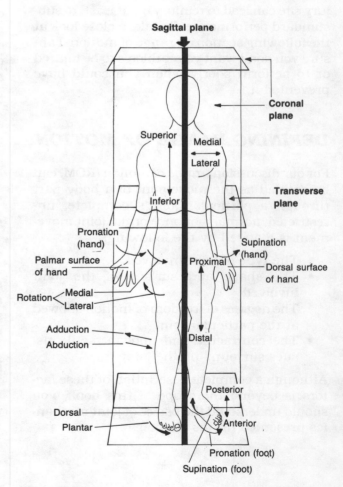

Figure 9.2. Primary planes of the body and the terms used to describe body movements and positions.

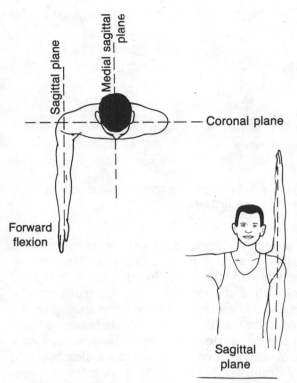

Figure 9.3. Active shoulder flexion occurring in the sagittal plane.

normal physiological motion would not be possible.

As in the example of shoulder flexion, in physiological flexion the arm is voluntarily moved overhead, and the humerus rolls and glides downward in the shoulder cavity (glenoid) to allow the arm to be raised fully overhead. Normal accessory motions are necessary for full, active physiological motion. Accessory motions can be performed by a trained sports medicine specialist to help restore normal motion. This is called joint mobilization and is discussed later.

PRINCIPLES OF RANGE OF MOTION

A thorough description of each motion available at a given joint is not vital and therefore is not presented in this book. Many fine kinesiology textbooks are available if additional information is desired. But a basic understanding of these joint movements will help you determine the mechanisms of common injury, appropriate therapeutic exercise interventions, and proper assessment procedures.

Prime Movers and Secondary Movers

The muscle primarily responsible for a given motion at a joint is called the *prime mover*. Muscles that assist the prime mover in the motion are the *secondary movers*. So, for a joint to move, the primary and the secondary movers must contract, generate enough force to overcome internal and external resistance, and then move the body segment on which they are inserted.

Agonists and Antagonists

Primary and secondary movers that produce physiological joint motion through muscular contraction are called *agonists*. Muscles located on the opposite side of the joint of the agonists are called *antagonists*. When an antagonist contracts, it produces movement opposite that of the agonist. Normal active motion requires controlled lengthening and relaxation of the antagonist to allow the agonist to produce desired joint motion. If the antagonistic muscle group is pathologically shortened or unable to relax to allow the agonist to produce sufficient force, normal ROM is restricted.

Flexibility

The neurological basis behind the principles of stretching is too complex to be discussed here. But, so that you understand how decreased flexibility relates to injury and how flexibility can be improved, I must introduce a few basics on flexibility.

Collagen

Soft tissue is one of the primary factors that limits abnormal motion and that most directly affects motion at a given joint. Healthy muscle tissue, however, does not play a significant role in flexibility. Rather, noncontractile connective tissue, or *collagen*, plays a more important part by providing most of the restraint to abnormal motion. It also restricts normal motion when flexibility is less than adequate.

Thus, attempts to increase ROM (flexibility) will be successful only if the following mechanical properties of collagen are addressed:

- Elasticity
- Viscoelasticity
- Plasticity

Elasticity

Collagen exhibits elastic properties. *Elasticity* refers to the principle whereby a load placed on tissue stretches that tissue to a degree dictated by the load; when the load is removed, the tissue returns to its preloaded length.

A good example of elasticity is a rubber band, which, when stretched to a point of tension and then released, returns to its original length.

Viscoelasticity

The *viscoelasticity* of collagen allows tissue to be stretched, depending on the load placed on the tissue due to the fluidlike (viscous) property of collagen. When the load is removed, the tissue does not immediately return to the preloaded state because of collagen's viscous property. This incomplete change in length, however, is not permanent. Eventually, the elastic component of collagen restores the tissue to its preloaded state.

Plasticity

The plastic component of collagen must be addressed for permanent change in collagen to occur. The stretchability of collagen allows for a permanent improvement in flexibility.

ASSESSING RANGE OF MOTION

Tools to assess ROM span from the simple use of the goniometer and tape measure to sophisticated electrogoniometers and digitized motion analysis. Perhaps the most common method of measuring joint motion is with a *goniometer*. This device is aligned with the bones of the joint, then its axis is aligned with the joint's axis of motion.

To evaluate AROM, you must ask the athlete to voluntarily move the joint through its full ROM. For PROM the joint is moved passively through the available ROM either by the examiner or by some other passive means. The corresponding angle of joint movement is observed on the goniometer (see Figure 9.4).

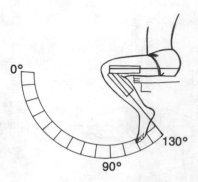

Figure 9.4. Goniometric measurement of active knee flexion.

In some cases, ROM can be assessed by a tape measure. This assessment also is particularly useful when gauging motion of the spinal column. Forward flexion of the trunk can be expressed as the distance from the tip of the fingers to the floor as the athlete bends forward at the waist. Be careful here, however, as your efforts to determine lower back flexibility in this manner may also be a function of hamstring length. Lateral flexion (or side bending) can be recorded as the distance the fingers are able to extend past the level of the knee joint as the athlete leans fully to one side and then the other. Extension can be measured as the distance from a given vertebral segment to a stationary point on the athlete's sacrum as he or she bends backward at the waist as far as possible.

NORMAL RESTRICTIONS ON RANGE OF MOTION

Several factors may restrict an athlete's ROM. In this section, I divide these factors into normal and abnormal categories. Uninjured athletes will typically encounter normal ROM restrictions, whereas injured athletes encounter both normal and abnormal restrictions.

Normal Restrictions on ROM

Joint movement is restricted at the end of the normal ROM for a particular joint by the following factors:

- Bone-to-bone contact
- Soft-tissue approximation
- Soft-tissue stiffness

Bone-to-Bone Contact

Some joints are normally restricted from abnormal motion when the two bones making up the joint contact each other. For example, when the elbow is completely straightened (extension), the bones of the forearm (radius and ulna) contact the upper arm bone (humerus). The bones fit snugly together in this position, preventing abnormal movement of the elbow.

Soft-Tissue Approximation

Some joints are normally restricted from further motion by contacting soft tissue outside the joint. For example, knee bending (flexion) when lying on the stomach (prone) is limited by the calf muscles making contact with the muscles of the back of the thigh.

Soft-Tissue Stiffness

Still other joints are held within normal limits by soft-tissue shortening or tightening. These soft tissues are noncontractile, meaning they do not have the ability to contract. Noncontractile tissues, unlike muscle, do not generate forces that cause their ends to be brought closer to one another.

Examples of noncontractile tissues are joint capsules and ligaments surrounding a joint. Joint capsules are composed of a tough, fibrous tissue that encloses the joint. Because of the joint capsule's design and where it attaches to the bones of the joint, the capsule checks against excessive motion.

Soft tissue located outside the joint capsule operates the same way. Ligaments are non-

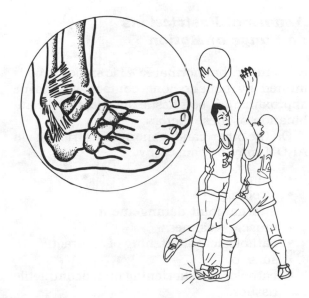

Figure 9.5. Lateral ligaments of the ankle helping to check excessive inversion.

contractile tissue outside the capsule that help to limit motion. The shape and attachment of ligaments at a particular joint check and restrict abnormal motion occurring at the joint. Figure 9.5 shows how abnormal motion (inversion) of the ankle is limited by ligaments.

Contractile tissue (muscle and tendon) also works with noncontractile soft tissue to prevent excessive joint motion. For example, the hip muscles help restrict motion of the hip joint (see Figure 9.6). Whereas the hip capsule tightens to provide primary restraint against excessive, abnormal motion, the front (anterior) hip muscles also provide some resistance to hyperextension.

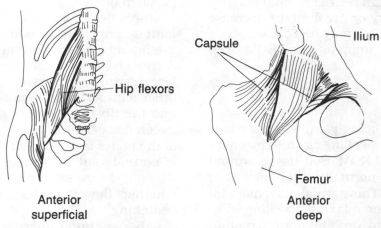

Figure 9.6. Hip flexor muscles (left) superficial to the anterior hip capsule (right) assist the capsule in checking hyperextension.

Abnormal Restrictions on Range of Motion

Remember that normal ROM is smooth and is limited by bone-to-bone contact, soft-tissue approximation, soft-tissue tightness, or a combination of these factors.

On the other hand, abnormal restrictions in AROM may be caused by

- pain,
- swelling,
- internal joint derangement,
- muscle weakness,
- pathological shortening of contractile tissues, or
- pathological shortening of noncontractile tissues.

Pain

Pain is nature's way of telling you that something is wrong. The sensation of pain helps to signal that things are out of normal synchrony. If moving a body part causes pain, the tendency is not to move it.

In addition, pain has a reflex effect on muscle. When pain is present, the involved muscle reflexively shuts down, and the contractile force of the muscle decreases. This reflex inhibition is muscle's response to pain resulting from injury to that muscle or related structures. After a time, normal muscle function will break down, causing muscle wasting, or *atrophy*. Prolonged pain and disuse produce additional muscle dysfunction. Finally, when muscle is rendered weak enough to affect its ability to generate sufficient force, the joint loses ROM.

Therefore, pain can restrict normal ROM by causing a voluntary or involuntary decrease in muscle activity. This may be a consequence of pain sensations stopping joint ROM or of reflex inhibition.

Swelling

In addition to producing pain, which we saw can decrease ROM, swelling can also mechanically block normal ROM. Soft tissue around a joint must move normally if the joint is to have normal ROM. This normal movement includes stretching and relaxing. Swelling within the soft tissue may prohibit normal motion by decreasing the ability of the soft tissues to smoothly stretch.

Another way in which swelling can decrease motion is when fluid is released into a joint as a result of injury. Such a fluid buildup is common in injuries to the anterior cruciate ligament of the knee (see Figure 9.7). This injury is prevalent in sports today and is discussed in great detail in chapter 11. The anterior cruciate ligament is a vascular structure that bleeds when its fibers are damaged; the blood escapes into the knee joint. If the joint capsule remains intact, the blood accumulates within the joint space, much like water fills a balloon. When the bleeding stops, the blood is held within the joint (hemarthrosis) by the intact joint capsule.

In a previously healthy knee, fluid within the joint usually indicates cruciate damage. Because the blood takes up space that is not usually occupied, normal motion is prevented by this excess fluid in the joint. And fluid within the knee joint also causes reflex inhibition of the quadriceps, compounding even further the decrease in ROM. Thus, if one of your athletes experiences knee swelling within 6 hours after injury, you should see that the athlete is cared for by a sports medicine specialist immediately.

Internal Joint Derangement

Internal joint derangement is the nonspecific description given to an injury of unknown extent to a structure within a joint. Although commonly used as a clinical diagnosis, internal joint derangement does not adequately describe any one injury. In this book, internal joint derangement refers to those cases in which some structure within a given joint is injured.

Again using the anterior cruciate tear as an example, let's look at one way that internal joint derangement can limit joint ROM. With the ligament torn, normal continuity is lost. A free end of the ligament, if both long and large enough, can become trapped between other joint structures, in this case the femur and the tibia. With the ligament caught between these bones, the normal gliding motion of the bones is prohibited. The result is a loss of normal joint mechanics and ROM. That is why physicians ask athletes with joint injuries whether they have experienced any joint "catching" or "locking."

Other common internal derangements resulting in decreased joint motion include cartilage (menisci) injuries of the knee, cartilage

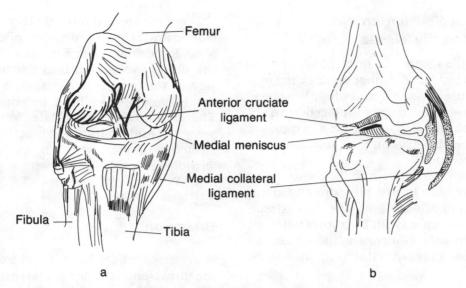

Figure 9.7. a, Intact anterior cruciate ligament; b, torn anterior cruciate ligament.

(labrum) injuries of the shoulder, and fragments of bone from intraarticular fractures.

Muscle Weakness

Muscles must be sufficiently strong for a joint to move actively through its full ROM. Considering the tremendous feats accomplished in athletics, this simple task would not seem difficult. However, the ability to move a body part against gravity requires a high degree of neuromuscular control, smooth activation of the primary and secondary muscles responsible for the motion, and synchrony between agonistic and antagonistic muscles. These principles are discussed in detail later in this chapter.

Pathological Shortening of Contractile Tissues

Contractile tissues are muscle-tendon units, which consist of the tendinous muscle origin, the muscle belly, and the tendinous insertion of the muscle. As a muscle contracts, it shortens and causes its site of attachment to move toward its origin (see Figure 9.8).

Pathological shortening of contractile tissue may be caused by prolonged immobilization of a joint, scarring of muscle, failure of the length of muscle to keep up with the rate of adjacent long-bone growth, excessive muscle tone (hypertonicity) caused by central nervous system dysfunction, and other muscular and neurological factors.

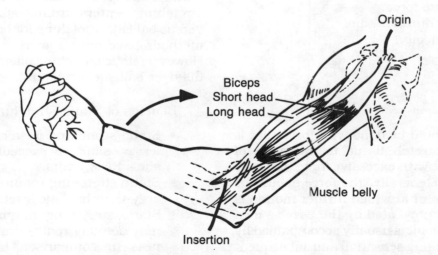

Figure 9.8. Muscle action. With the hand freely mobile, elbow flexion occurs as the prime mover's (biceps) insertions move toward the muscle's origin.

Pathological Shortening of Noncontractile Tissue

Noncontractile tissue can be stretched by external forces but alone cannot produce the tension that causes tissue shortening. However, if a noncontractile structure is placed in an abnormally shortened position for a prolonged period of time, the structure will maintain that shortened position.

Shortening of noncontractile tissue commonly occurs after injury, after prolonged immobilization of a joint, and when soft-tissue length fails to keep up with the rate of adjacent long-bone growth. Noncontractile tissue, as you will see, plays a vital role in overall flexibility.

DEVELOPING A STRETCHING PROGRAM

Now that you understand the components of normal ROM, the basic methods of assessing motion, and the factors that limit ROM, let's examine how you can design a program that will effectively address your athletes' ROM limitations. Then, before actually designing a stretching program for your athletes, refer to Appendix A for appropriate guidelines.

Optimizing gains in flexibility requires that the involved noncontractile tissue undergo a deforming force. However, this force must be applied in a safe, efficient manner. That's why all effective stretching programs include exercises of

- appropriate force,
- adequate duration, and
- proper velocity.

Force

Stretching should be done with force that is adequate to stretch tissue to the point of benefit but not with excessive force that may cause injury. Generally, the force should be applied to a point at which further motion is limited, being prevented by the tissue's own tension. This point is usually accompanied by a moderate pulling sensation and subsequent relaxation.

Properly applied force will stress the visco-elastic and plastic properties of collagen and allow force relaxation. Excessive force beyond the pulling sensation into the painful range signals the muscle to contract, which defeats the purpose of stretching: to lengthen tissues. Therefore, the appropriate force must be achieved and maintained whether an athlete stretches alone, with an assisting device (crutches, cane, etc.), or with a partner.

Duration

Many researchers have sought to determine the most efficient length of time a stretch should be held. Their results show that 6- to 30-second stretches are beneficial for gaining flexibility. Generally speaking, to maintain flexibility, a shorter duration of stretching is sufficient.

Another consideration is how often athletes should stretch. Again, daily stretching maintains flexibility; but, to increase flexibility, stretching twice a day or more is necessary.

Finally, the athlete must increase the amount of force in addition to duration and frequency. For example, a daily set of efficient, aggressive stretches will yield greater results than stretching two or three times a day with less than adequate force and duration.

Velocity

Perhaps the greatest controversy concerning stretching centers around static stretching versus ballistic stretching (or bouncing). Both methods have been shown to be beneficial. However, static stretching offers distinct benefits over ballistic stretching.

Benefits of Static Stretching

- Static stretching is safer, offering less possibility of exceeding the tissue's ROM limits.
- Static stretching requires less energy than ballistic stretching.
- Static stretching minimizes and may actually reduce muscle soreness in comparison to ballistic stretching.

That is not to say that ballistic stretching plays no role in a proper stretching program for the athlete. Because most athletic events are ballistic in nature, athletes must be able to perform these movements safely. However, strict guidelines for ballistic stretching must be adhered to by athletes. Ballistic stretching should be performed only after adequate warm-up and static stretching. And ballistic stretching should be confined to small ROMs, or just past the motion attained with normal static stretching (no greater than 10% past the normal static range).

RANGE OF MOTION GOALS

Rehabilitation goals of the acute phase are to

- maintain ROM,
- get sufficient rest, and
- protect the involved body part from further injury.

Goals of the subacute phase are to

- reestablish normal ROM and
- regain muscle strength.

The primary goal of the chronic phase is to

- reestablish normal flexibility.

Additional ROM Concerns

In addition to the force, duration, and velocity of stretching exercises, other factors play important roles in a sound stretching program.

Muscle Temperature

As collagen is heated, the force required to gain or maintain a given tissue length decreases. However, laboratory findings inconsistently support the idea that heating muscles will increase joint movement. But in some cases elevated tissue temperature and stretching can yield greater gains in flexibility than can stretching used alone.

Overstretching

Stretching is a key component in athletic rehabilitation and function. However, excessive stretching is counterproductive. So, how do you know when your athletes are stretching too much?

To monitor the extent of stretching, observe your athletes and answer the following questions:

- During the stretch, is there involuntary muscle quivering or shaking?
- During the stretch, is pain present?
- During the stretch, are form and coordination maintained?
- Does pain increase after stretching?
- Is ROM decreased after stretching?

Proper Form

Position of the body part is vital if stretching is to be successful. The joint stretched should be aligned with the connective tissues stressed. All joints crossed by a muscle group involved in the stretch must be arranged appropriately. When pain or excessive tightness prevents effective stretching of a two-joint muscle at each joint, then one joint should be stressed at a time. One sign that the stretch is excessive is that the athlete will voluntarily or involuntarily use improper form.

Hypermobility

Some athletes are hypermobile; that is, they exhibit too much joint motion. Tall, thin athletes (ectomorphs) commonly exhibit this trait. Female athletes tend to be more hypermobile than males. However, this trait is certainly not restricted to a given body type or sex. Simple screening methods performed by trained staff can determine excessive joint play. In cases of generalized hypermobility, aggressive stretching may need to be avoided or at least deemphasized.

However, certain sports stress body parts uniquely, and hypermobility of these joints is not considered abnormal. For example, consider the unique external rotation of the shoulder required by a baseball pitcher.

Individual Response

Each athlete is unique, responding in a unique way to various modes of stretching. Individual differences must be taken into account. The athlete's response to the program dictates the optimum protocol to follow.

General Guidelines for a Successful Stretching Program

1. Begin with gentle warm-up activities, such as brisk walking, light jogging, or calisthenics, to elevate muscle temperature. When appropriate, 20 minutes of moist heat applied to a particular area before stretching may be of some benefit.

2. Follow with one set of 15 repetitions of static stretches, maintaining a hold for 8 to 10 seconds at the point of gentle discomfort.

3. After static stretching, gentle ballistic stretching may be executed at all noninjured joints for one set of 10 repetitions at a length no greater than 10% of normal static stretching length.

4. Practice, functional progression, or strengthening work should be done at this time (after warm-up and static stretching). If the athlete is competing, ballistic stretching (if tolerated) of the involved joint should be done after warm-up and static stretching.

5. More vigorous stretching should follow athletic activity, when elevated tissue temperature will facilitate prolonged stretching. Athletes should perform two sets of 15 static stretches, each for 20 to 30 seconds. Ice may be used after the previous steps until the injured area is numb.

6. To facilitate greater gains in flexibility, this program may be repeated later the same day when done in conjunction with rehabilitation. Exercises to increase ROM can be done three or four times a day.

7. Prolonged static stretching for 10 to 15 minutes may also be practically incorporated into a daily routine. Calf muscles are stretched effectively with a slant board in the same way that hamstrings are stretched against a wall. For a guide to stretching movements, the structures being stretched, and common substitutions, refer to Appendix A.

RANGE OF MOTION EXERCISE RESTRICTIONS AND RECOMMENDATIONS

The type of ROM exercises and the intensity with which they are performed are determined, in large part, by the injured athlete's stage of rehabilitation.

Acute-Phase Exercise Restrictions

Immediately after injury, ROM at a particular joint may be restricted. During the acute phase of athlete rehabilitation, pain and swelling are the primary restrictions on normal ROM. Until the exact nature of the injury, the degree of involvement, and the specific structures involved are known, joint movement should be avoided. The carefully selected active and passive movements to assist in the diagnosis of injury should be left to a trained specialist.

Gentle, active motion within the pain-free range can be started soon after injury. The less severe the injury, the sooner motion can be started. Both AAROM and PROM after acute injury help to decrease swelling, promote healing, maintain soft-tissue pliability, and nourish joint cartilage.

However, if an athlete experiences pain with motion, AROM, AAROM, and PROM should be avoided, especially in the first few days after injury. Motion that reproduces the way in

---

Therapeutic ROM exercise in the acute phase must be pain free, must not be forced, and must not cause an increase in swelling.

which the injury was initially sustained also should be avoided.

Overzealous AAROM and PROM can cause more local bleeding or further damage injured tissue, thereby compounding the problem. A good way to judge whether motion is detrimental is to see whether it causes pain during the motion or an increase in swelling after the motion.

Active muscle movement is actually the best way to move the fluid that builds up at the injury site. And gentle AROM combined with compression is probably the most effective means to decrease swelling. But excessive motion before the injury is resolved will produce greater swelling. Thus, in the early stages after injury, these ROM exercise guidelines should be followed:

- No motion should be allowed until the injury is carefully evaluated.
- So that possible further injury is prevented, motion should never be forced.
- Avoid PROM, especially in the hands of an untrained individual.
- Active-assisted ROM must be done in a controlled manner, with no excessive assistance.
- Active ROM should be performed in a pain-free range.
- Active ROM should be performed with the involved body part elevated, as this will facilitate efforts to decrease swelling.

Acute-Phase ROM Exercises

The following section describes some specific exercises that may be done during the acute phase of injury. Each of the exercises should be performed in accordance with the ROM exercise guidelines listed in the previous section.

Neck (Cervical Spine)

Athletes (especially those in contact sports) who do not have full ROM of the neck are candidates for serious injury. Insufficient ROM cannot adequately dissipate forces through the cervical spine. These forces, if strong enough, can cause catastrophic spinal cord and peripheral nerve damage. Full AROM of the neck is shown in Figure 9.9.

The neck should be immobilized after acute injury if nerve damage is suspected or if the weight of the head stresses the injured tissue

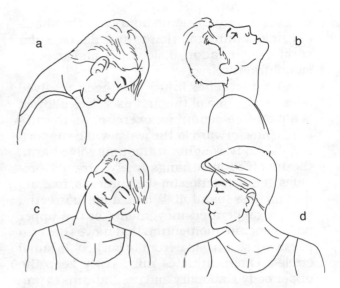

Figure 9.9. Active ROM of the cervical spine: a, flexion; b, extension; c, left lateral flexion; d, right rotation.

sufficiently to cause increased muscle spasm and pain.

> No painful active motion and no passive motion of the cervical spine should be performed until involvement of the spine has been ruled out.

Midrange AROM is allowed only if it is pain free. Forward flexion can be started if it does not cause pain, numbness, or tingling in the arms. Rotation to the right and left is also usually encouraged early. Lateral flexion may also be started in the acute phase, again depending on whether it causes pain. Lateral flexion is especially effective for stretching the upper trapezius muscle. If this motion is tolerated without pain or spasm, it can greatly help in loosening up the neck.

Care should be taken in those athletes suffering from symptoms after a brachial plexus stretch (burner or stinger). Extension, especially with rotation and lateral flexion, causes the vertebrae to closely approximate one another and should be avoided if bony pathology or nerve-root irritation is suspected.

Shoulder and Shoulder Girdle

The shoulder and shoulder girdle are commonly affected in both acute and chronic sport injuries. Common acute injuries of the shoulder (glenohumeral) joint include capsular sprain, subluxation, dislocation, and an occasional fracture.

After the acute injury has been resolved adequately, one of the first exercises allowed is a pain-free pendulum exercise. As the athlete bends forward at the waist while supporting the body weight on the uninvolved arm, the involved arm hangs freely. Gravity provides gentle traction on the humerus, making motion less painful. When done correctly, these exaggerated movements of the upper body generate momentum that moves the arm passively side to side, front to back, or in small circles. Often, athletes mistakenly keep the upper body stationary and use the arms to produce the desired motion. However, this pulls the head of the humerus back toward the shoulder joint, minimizing traction placed on the joint.

If the athlete's arm is in a sling, the forearm should be removed from the sling throughout the day to allow for pain-free active motion at the elbow.

Elbow, Wrist, and Hand

The most frequent acute injuries of the wrist and elbow in sport are fractures and dislocations. Particularly common in contact sports are posterior elbow dislocations and wrist and hand fractures. Acute strains, sprains, tendon ruptures, and contusions are also common in contact sports.

Range of motion exercises for these structures are essential following the postinjury immobilization period. Uninvolved body parts may be removed from protective immobilization and stressed by the athlete through pain-free ROM throughout the day. Motion, in conjunction with elevation, will effectively reduce swelling.

Athletes with conditions that do not require immobilization but that do require restricted activity should engage in pain-free AROM activities with the involved structures. Motion of the elbow should address flexion and extension as well as pronation and supination (see Figure 9.10). Similarly, the wrist should be moved within pain-free limits in flexion, extension, and radial and ulnar deviation (see Figure 9.11). Also recommended are grasping activities, finger straightening and bending, and thumb movements toward and away from the palm and toward the fingertips.

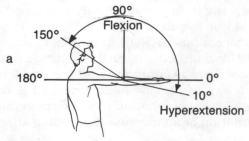

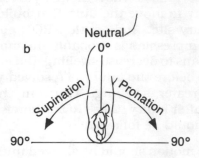

Elbow pronation and supination

Figure 9.10. Active elbow ROM: a, flexion and extension; b, pronation and supination.

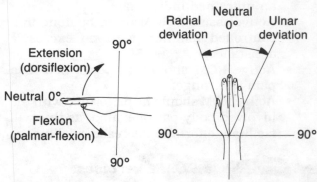

Wrist flexion and extension Radial and ulnar deviation
a b

Figure 9.11. Active wrist ROM: a, flexion and extension; and b, radial and ulnar deviation.

Upper and Lower Back

Acute injuries to the upper back (thoracic spine) are rare but usually involve muscle strains when they do occur. Injuries to the lower back (lumbar spine) are more frequent.

When acute lower back injury occurs, it is vital to examine carefully the sensation and muscle function of the legs to rule out spinal cord or nerve-root involvement. Once bone, disk, and nerve-root damage have been ruled out, the resultant muscle spasm must be addressed. Muscular and ligament sprains often respond to rest, modalities, medication, and generic exercise programs. However, a therapeutic exercise program that specifically addresses the injured area may produce a quicker, more complete recovery.

Often, rest is indicated for serious acute soft-tissue injury of the back. Rest for acute back injury entails decreased activity, even to the point of bed rest. But lower back injuries are often rested too long, especially when pain-free ROM would decrease pain and stiffness.

Traditional flexion exercises consisting of AAROM and PROM knee-to-chest activities are especially effective in the acute phase when done in the pain-free midrange. Also helpful are hook-lying (rotation) exercises, which facilitate muscle relaxation (see Figure 9.12).

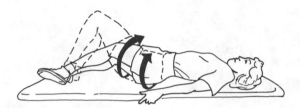

Figure 9.12. Hook-lying rotation. The athlete flexes at the hips and knees, keeping the feet flat and the knees together. The legs are allowed to fall to one side to the point of gentle discomfort. The exercise is then repeated to the opposite side.

Flexion postures and activities are contraindicated in the case of a potential ruptured disk, whereas extension positions have been shown to benefit such injuries. These extension activities also should be actively assisted and performed to midrange. Active extension is contraindicated in the case of an acute sprain or strain of the lower back.

Hip, Pelvis, and Groin

Hip, pelvic, and groin injuries are not as prevalent as other lower extremity injuries. But acute injury to the muscles around the hip, pelvic, and groin regions can easily become chronic if not properly treated. Treatment of these regions consists of isolated stretching of the involved soft tissues.

For example, a pulled groin is best identified and rehabilitated by isolating the hip flexors and the hip adductors (see Figure 9.13). Then, stretches that specifically address the involved muscle group can be prescribed and performed.

Acute injuries of the hip and pelvis include the infrequent but catastrophic hip disloca-

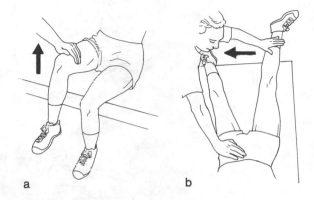

a   b

Figure 9.13. Ways to isolate hip flexor and adductor involvement by applying manual resistance: a, testing hip flexors; b, testing hip adductors.

tion; the hip pointer, a painful bruise of the iliac crest; and an avulsion fracture of the pelvis. Athletes experiencing extreme tenderness on or around the pelvis must be X-rayed. If walking is painful and cannot be done normally (no limp) and at a typical cadence, an assisting device should be used.

When appropriate, the athlete can begin pain-free midrange hip flexion, extension, abduction, and adduction, as well as internal and external rotation activities (see Figure 9.14). Extreme ROM should be avoided, especially if it is painful or if the movement reproduces that by which the injury was initially sustained.

Knee

Perhaps no other joint in the body has received more attention from sports medicine specialists than the knee. As a result, tremendous gains have been made in the evaluation and treatment of knee injuries. Knowledge of particular knee injuries has helped make commonplace the accurate assessment of most sport-related knee injuries.

Rule changes in contact and collision sports have helped to decrease the incidence of traumatic knee injuries. Conditioning, agility, and flexibility programs have also helped reduce the occurrence of knee injuries in particular sports. However, the knee joint remains the most frequently injured joint in sport.

The knee rehabilitation process should begin when diagnostic and treatment measures have been completed. Depending on the type and severity of knee injury, ROM activities may be permitted or may be absolutely contraindicated.

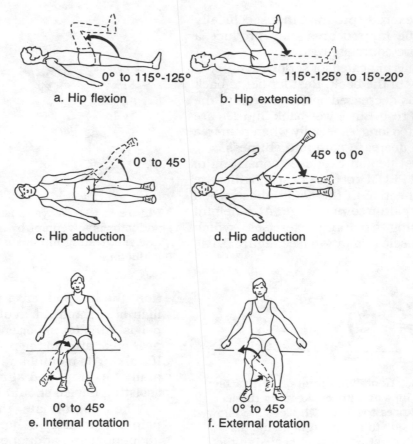

a. Hip flexion   0° to 115°-125°

b. Hip extension   115°-125° to 15°-20°

c. Hip abduction   0° to 45°

d. Hip adduction   45° to 0°

e. Internal rotation   0° to 45°

f. External rotation   0° to 45°

Figure 9.14.   Active hip ROM.

If a knee injury results in any of the following conditions, no attempts at vigorous motion should be made, and the appropriate sports medicine specialist should be consulted:

• Restricted ROM
• Swelling within 12 hours
• Locking or catching sensations

Pain-free knee flexion (bending) is usually permitted in the acute phase. This motion should be performed to midrange in either an active-assisted or a passive manner. Common methods of active-assisted knee flexion are shown in Figure 9.15.

Acute-phase treatment of muscle injury to the quadriceps or hamstrings should vary according to the severity of the condition. Minor strains may allow gentle AAROM in the pain-free midrange; but the strained muscle must not be stretched to stressful ROM limits.

Moderate and severe strains may warrant complete rest throughout the acute phase. An assisting device should be used for walking until the gait is performed pain free, without deviation, and the affected knee is able to bear full weight with no increase in swelling.

Calf, Ankle, and Foot

The lower leg and foot regions are particularly susceptible to sport injury. In fact, injury-rate studies of certain sports have found that ankle sprains occur even more frequently than knee injuries. In addition, overuse injuries of the calf, ankle, and foot are quite common in runners and other athletes who run, jog, sprint, and jump. And fractures of the long bones of the lower leg and acute soft-tissue damage to the calf are also not unusual consequences of sport participation.

The two most common acute calf injuries are Achilles tendon ruptures and tears of the inner (medial) head of the gastrocnemius muscle ("tennis leg"). Achilles tendon rupture

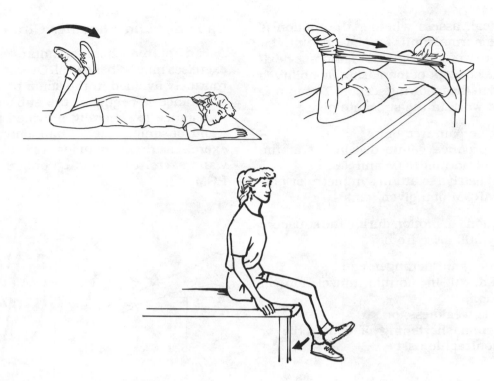

Figure 9.15.   Active-assisted knee flexion.

is sometimes confused with ankle injury; so, if you are at all uncertain about an injury to that area, refer the athlete to an orthopedist immediately. When the acute symptoms of medial gastrocnemius strain have subsided, dorsiflexion of the ankle is beneficial in increasing ROM and decreasing swelling. All active plantar flexion should be pain free. Other ankle motions are usually not involved (inversion and eversion) and can usually be stressed acutely.

Most ankle sprains are inversion sprains, involving the anterior talofibular ligament. In such cases, gentle AROM or AAROM dorsiflexion, plantar flexion, and eversion are helpful. These ankle motions and active toe motions with elevation also may decrease swelling. Other active motions that may be beneficial include ankle circles or tracing the letters of the alphabet with the big toe.

Eversion ankle sprains can be more involved than inversion sprains and take even longer to rehabilitate. The same general principles apply, however, in that all ROM exercises should be pain free. If the athlete cannot walk without pain when bearing full weight on the affected side in a normal gait sequence, an assisting device should be used.

Subacute-Phase Exercise Restrictions

The subacute phase of injury typically refers to the period of time between the acute phase (up to 72 hours after the injury is sustained) and the chronic phase (from 6 months to 1 year). But, because the status of an injury can change dramatically during this time, the subacute phase is referred to as the time the initial injury begins to resolve itself until AROM of the affected joint is symmetrical with the uninvolved side. Restrictions on ROM during the subacute phase stem from the aftereffects of rest (i.e., soft-tissue tightness and muscle weakness).

When the back and the neck are involved, the subacute phase lasts until motion on each side of the joint axis is normal and symmetrical (e.g., the degree of side bending is the same to the right as it is to the left).

Pain, swelling, and other symptoms of acute injury should be resolved in the subacute phase. The athlete should have pain-free joint ROM when engaged in light exercise activities. Rehabilitation efforts during the subacute phase should try to achieve functional symmetry between the affected side and the side that is not injured. As soon as motion is symmetrical, assess whether the motion is within the normal limits for a given joint. If it is not, more work is required to improve flexibility. The concept of increasing flexibility is addressed in the following section. To summarize, ROM work in the subacute phase

- must be pain free but
- may produce gentle discomfort at the ends of normal ROM and
- should strive to attain symmetry or normal AROM of a given joint.

Restrictions in motion during the subacute stage may still arise from

- internal joint derangement,
- breakdown in normal muscle-tendon function,
- muscle weakness, or
- abnormal shortening of contractile or noncontractile tissue.

Subacute-Phase ROM Exercises

In the subacute phase, exercises should emphasize AROM through the full range. Gentle, passive overpressure or active-assisted motion at the end of the range is allowed during the subacute phase. Once ROM is pain free and symmetrical, more aggressive work to regain muscle strength takes precedence over ROM work.

Neck (Cervical Spine)

In keeping with the subacute-phase goals to normalize and make symmetrical the athletes's joint motion, you should make sure that AROM neck exercises are addressed in all planes. For equal rotation and lateral flexion to the left and the right, gentle manual overpressure at the ends of ROM may prove beneficial. For example, to enhance lateral flexion, the athlete should simply rest the hand on top of the head, letting the weight of the arm gently assist the ear toward the shoulder.

> All AAROM exercises involving the neck should be pain free. And you should never force motion of the neck by pulling down on the head.

Shoulder and Shoulder Girdle

As an injured shoulder improves, AAROM exercises may be beneficial. Overhead motions routinely avoided in the acute phase require assistance if begun in the subacute phase. Assistance is generally provided by a cane, wand, or similar object. Commonly used wand exercises are shown in Figure 9.16. Midrange wand exercises should be progressed to full ROM.

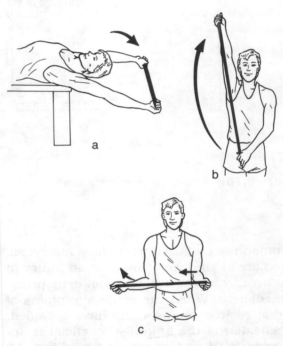

Figure 9.16. Active-assisted shoulder ROM: a, supine flexion; b, standing abduction; c, standing external rotation.

Care should be taken at the ends of ROM, especially when flexing and abducting the shoulder after acromioclavicular injury or impingement syndrome of the rotator cuff. Abduction should also be watched carefully in combination with external rotation when anterior shoulder dislocations are being rehabilitated. Pulley systems are also helpful in overhead AAROM work.

Elbow, Wrist, and Hand

Active-assisted ROM activities for the elbow, wrist, and hand are best performed with the assistance of the opposite (uninvolved) arm. When assisting finger motion either actively or passively, force should be applied lightly, preferably with only one finger from the opposite hand.

Two conditions that warrant special care in the subacute phase are deep bruises to the upper arm and navicular fractures. Deep upper arm contusions that involve the brachialis (biceps) muscle should not be actively or passively forced into elbow extension. The reason for caution is that the brachialis has a tendency to bleed, and the escaped blood may calcify in the muscle belly, a condition called *myositis ossificans*. Deep upper arm contusions should be referred for special rehabilitation to minimize the risk of developing this condition. The notorious navicular fracture is a common injury to the wrist that usually results from a fall onto a hyperextended wrist. Such fractures are often undetected because X rays taken at the time of injury read negative. And because the navicular bone has a poor blood supply, complications often arise in the healing process. Even when acute symptoms do subside, active-assisted and passive extension to the extremes of motion should be avoided.

Upper and Lower Back

Active-assisted ROM can be progressed through all planes to the ends of ROM if the athlete experiences no pain. Hamstrings and hip flexors should be of particular concern as these muscles often contribute to lower back problems. A careful analysis of those muscles may be warranted, especially for chronic or recurring back conditions. If tolerated, the hamstrings, hip flexors, and their related structures should be stretched carefully during the subacute phase.

Hip, Pelvis, and Groin

Single-joint movement of the hips and pelvis to the ends of ROM can begin when the motion causes no pain. However, many muscles around the hip cross two joints (hip and knee), so you must see that athletes begin stretching at one joint only before they progress to the second joint. And, when stretching the muscles of the hip and pelvis in a skeletally immature athlete, you must make sure that the muscle does not pull its bony attachment away from the pelvis, which will aggravate an avulsion fracture.

Knee

In general, flexion and icing of the knee often aid rehabilitation efforts in the subacute phase. If athletes can tolerate it, active-assisted and passive knee flexion should progress through the available ROM. Gentle, assisted extension movements may also proceed if motion is smooth and pain free. Persistent limitations in extension in the subacute phase may indicate severe cartilage or ligament damage. And, never force knee extension if pain is felt by the athlete.

Isolated single-joint stretching of the quadriceps and hamstrings, first at the knee and then at the hip, is an effective exercise for subacute-phase strains. However, deep thigh contusions to the quadriceps must be very carefully addressed because the quadriceps tend to bleed excessively after severe contusion or tearing, and, like the brachialis muscle, myositis ossificans could result. Overzealous stretching of the quadriceps may produce more bleeding and compound the process. Therefore, the rehabilitation of deep quadriceps contusions should be left to a sports medicine specialist.

Calf, Ankle, Foot

Calf strain treatment during the subacute phase should involve progressive stretching of the gastrocnemius and soleus muscle groups. The stretching movements can progress from active-assisted to carefully controlled passive work.

Approaches to the management of ankle sprains vary, ranging from aggressive, early mobilization to surgery. During the subacute phase, dorsiflexion of the ankle is beneficial. Later, dorsiflexion can be combined with plantar flexion and the motion involved in the initial injury to return the ankle to normal, symmetrical ROM.

Chronic-Phase Exercise Restrictions

The chronic phase of injury typically refers to a period of time from 6 months to 1 year. Rehabilitation efforts, if undertaken, usually fall short of attaining normal sport-specific ROM. If formal rehabilitation efforts have been undertaken, symmetrical ROM with the opposite side often is the goal, and that is where ROM efforts stop. For our purposes, therefore, I consider the chronic phase to be after AROM of the unaffected area is symmetrical with the opposite side. When the neck and back are involved, the chronic phase begins after symmetry of motion is present on both sides of the joint axis.

During the chronic phase, the primary restriction to normal ROM is inadequate length of contractile or noncontractile tissue. Many factors contribute to such restrictions: poor posture, unhealthy daily living habits, improper sport-specific training habits, or inadequate muscle strength on the opposite side of the joint.

Chronic-Phase ROM Exercises

The manifestation of chronic sport injury can often be traced to inadequate management of the problem in the acute and subacute phases. Previous sections of this chapter addressed the proper ROM management of common sport injuries during these two phases. This background may help you prevent such problems from becoming chronic.

However, participation in sports in which the athlete is constantly striving to jump higher, run faster, or throw harder may result in chronic injury even if the injury is properly managed initially. In these cases, inadequate preinjury ROM is often a contributing factor. So let's look at specific ways that you can decrease the incidence of chronic sport injury on your team.

Neck (Cervical Spine)

Chronic limitations in cervical ROM should be thoroughly evaluated to rule out involvement of the spine, especially in athletes involved in contact sports. Postural abnormalities commonly manifest as chronic abnormal motion. In the cervical region, a forward head posture is typified by the overall forward-thrusting appearance of the head (see Figure 9.17). This

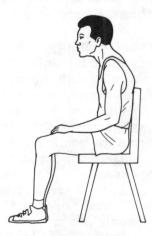

Figure 9.17. Exaggerated forward head posture.

condition is especially common in the adolescent athlete and may play a role in muscle tightness and headaches at the base of the skull and aching in the neck.

A simple way to assess this is to look at your athlete from the side. If you were to draw an imaginary line through the ear to the bottom of the earlobe, this line should meet the tip of the shoulder. If this imaginary line falls in front of the tip of the shoulder, then a forward head posture is present.

The reverse of this position, the flat neck posture, is a good postural exercise and may help decrease chronic pain in this area (see Figure 9.18).

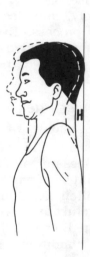

Figure 9.18. Flat neck exercise.

Shoulder and Shoulder Girdle

Bursitis and tendinitis of the biceps and rotator cuff tendons may be acute but much more frequently are chronic. A common overuse injury of the shoulder involves the supraspinatus tendon, the biceps tendon, or both being pinched between the humerus and the corocoacromial ligament (a ligament in the front of the shoulder area). Athletes with this impingement syndrome often exhibit postural problems in addition to chronic pain.

For example, an athlete may be round shouldered in that the shoulders are in a forward position relative to the head (see Figure 9.19). The head and neck are in acceptable alignment, but the shoulders are well in front of the line running from the ear to the shoulder.

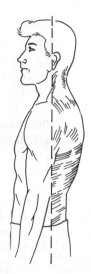

Figure 9.19. Forward shoulder posture.

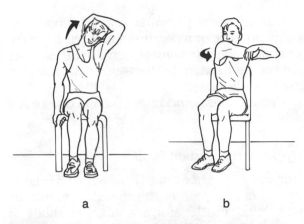

Figure 9.21. a, Stretching the right-side upper trapezius; b, stretching the right-side middle trapezius and rhomboids.

Elbow, Wrist, and Hand

A challenging problem involving the elbow is lateral epicondylitis, or tennis elbow. It is not unusual for this painful condition to last longer than a year. Flexibility of the elbow and wrist joints, as well as the tissue length of the involved muscles, must be maintained during prolonged healing, but not at the expense of increased pain. Therefore, elbow extension, forearm pronation and supination, and wrist flexion are recommended, but not if pain is experienced. Thus, athletes should isolate each motion before progressing to a combination of movements. These exercises will help maintain length of the lateral elbow muscles.

Round-shouldered athletes should perform exercises that stretch the pectorals (see Figure 9.20).

Chronic overuse, muscle flexibility imbalance, or an acute flare-up of pain from a chronic problem may all manifest as a clinical entity known as *myofascial pain syndrome*. This problem is characterized by dull aching interspersed with sharp pain. The pain may be localized at a so-called trigger point or at a site away from the main point of discomfort. Common muscles involved in myofascial pain syndrome are the trapezius, rhomboids, supraspinatus, infraspinatus, and levator scapulae. These muscles can be stretched to help alleviate myofascial pain (see Figure 9.21).

When medial epicondylitis occurs, elbow extension, forearm supination, and wrist extension are beneficial. Common among baseball pitchers, volleyball players, and football quarterbacks is medial overload syndrome of the elbow, in which ligamentous and muscular structures on the medial aspect of the elbow are repeatedly stressed. Although this condition primarily involves the ligamentous and capsular structures of the elbow, muscles in the arm may go into reflex protective spasms. Therefore, maintenance of wrist flexion and pronator flexibility is also important.

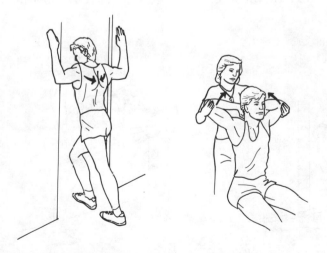

Figure 9.20. Pectoral stretching.

Before allowing adolescent athletes with medial overload syndrome ("Little League elbow") to engage in ROM activities for the elbow, you must be certain there is no avulsion fracture in the area.

Chronic wrist pain may result from a navicular fracture or a condition involving the triangular cartilage complex on the little-finger side of the wrist. In both cases, ROM exercises are of little benefit.

Chronic hand and finger pain is rare in the athlete.

Upper and Lower Back

Chronic upper back pain is most often related to myofascial pain of the rhomboids, middle trapezius, and levator scapulae. Methods to stretch these areas have already been presented (see pp. 84-85).

Overuse injuries of the back are common in athletes who perform repetitive hyperextension activities. Such athletes include offensive football linemen (pass blocking), gymnasts and dancers, and athletes who continuously run and jump on hard surfaces (indoor track and basketball). As the lower back is extended, the portions of the lumbar vertebrae that allow movement move close together. Hyperextension causes the vertebrae to close together tightly, stressing the structures even further. Repetitive hyperextension, because of the ongoing stress placed on the articular structures of the vertebrae, often results in stress fracture, for which extension, and especially hyperextension, is contraindicated.

Hip, Groin, and Pelvis

Many recurrent groin pulls result from inadequate flexibility or muscle flexibility imbalance on the opposite side of the hip joint. "Snapping hip" at the greater trochanter results from inadequate flexibility of the hip abductors. Runners often suffer chronic upper hamstring strain, which is characterized by pain at the buttocks during a run or stiffness in the same area after prolonged sitting. Inadequate flexibility of the hamstrings contributes to this chronic condition. I describe ways to stretch the hamstrings in the next section on the management of chronic knee problems.

Knee

An athlete's knee extension and flexion may be limited following significant ligamentous injury, even in its chronic phase. A significant loss of flexion (less than 110°) will make stair climbing, squatting, and other activities difficult. Obviously, such ligament damage to the knees should be checked thoroughly by a sports medicine specialist.

A lack of hamstring flexibility is inherent to many overuse injuries of the knee. It is especially prevalent during the adolescent growth spurt or in the otherwise sedentary recreational athlete and has a direct effect on recurrent hamstring strain and patellofemoral pain.

Patellofemoral pain is a more accurate description of a condition sometimes called *chondromalacia patellae*. Patellofemoral pain is characterized by dull aching around the kneecap and may be sharp at times (especially when going up or down stairs or when arising after prolonged sitting). Athletes can stretch their hamstrings and help avoid hamstring strains and patellofemoral pain by performing the exercises shown in Figure 9.22.

Hamstring flexibility can be easily assessed by having the athlete flex the hip to 90° while lying on the back (supine) and then actively extend the knee (see Figure 5.1, p. 34). An ath-

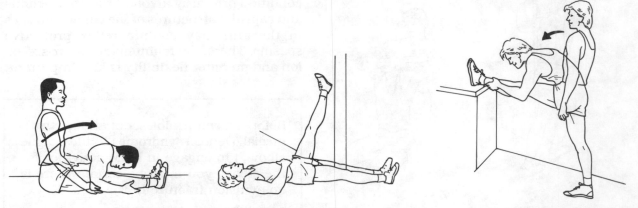

Figure 9.22.   Common methods to stretch the hamstrings.

lete should be able to straighten the knee to 10° or less.

On the other side of the joint, quadriceps tightness often contributes to recurrent quadriceps strain. Methods to stretch the quadriceps are shown in Figure 9.23.

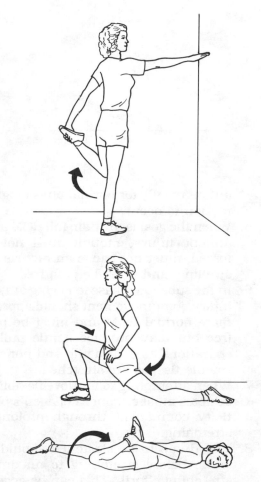

Figure 9.23. Common methods to stretch the quadriceps.

The lateral knee pain that is common in runners is often caused by inadequate length of the iliotibial band. Dull aching and occasional sharp pain along the outside of the knee are experienced as the iliotibial band slides over the femoral condyle during knee flexion and extension. Stretching the iliotibial band and tensor fascia lata helps manage this problem (see Figure 9.24).

Ankle, Calf, and Foot

Unfortunately, recurrent ankle sprains are commonly referred to our clinic. These

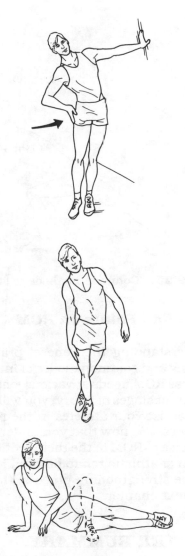

Figure 9.24. Common methods to stretch the iliotibial band.

chronic sprains usually have not regained preinjury flexibility, strength, and proprioception by the time athletes are allowed to return to full participation. (If only I had a dollar for every ankle sprain that was reinjured because of inadequate rehabilitation.)

Tightness of the gastrocnemius and soleus (calf) muscles is inherent both to many problems of the ankle and foot and to recurrent ankle sprains. Tight calves are also a major contributing factor in inflammation of the Achilles tendon and the plantar fascia, muscle overload of the front (anterior) calf muscles (anterior shin splints), and inflammation at the insertion of the Achilles tendon in the skeletally immature athlete (Sever's disease). Methods to stretch the calves are shown in Figure 9.25.

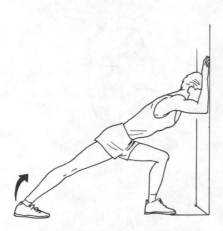
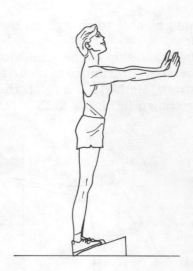
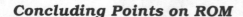

Figure 9.25.   Common methods to stretch the calves.

Concluding Points on ROM

By understanding the general principles of stretching and common modes of intervention to address ROM needs at various joints during the different stages of injury, you will be better able to assist your athletes in the rehabilitation process. So now that you understand the importance of ROM in the therapeutic exercise program of athletic rehabilitation, let's move on to the strengthening process, the subject of the next chapter.

CHAPTER SUMMARY

1. Adequate ROM is required for the full joint function and force generation needed in sport participation.
2. Abnormal ROM caused by pain, swelling, internal joint derangement, muscle weakness, or pathological shortening of contractile and noncontractile tissue is a major concern addressed in the sport rehabilitation process.
3. Range of motion is classified as being active (AROM), passive (PROM), or active assisted (AAROM).
4. Movements that an athlete chooses to perform are known as physiological motions. Accessory motions are movements that must occur naturally and automatically for normal physiological motion to occur.
5. When the goal is to attain full ROM after athletic injury, motion must not be forced, must not cause an increase in swelling, and must be pain free.
6. In the subacute phase following athletic injury, joint movement should approximate normal ROM and must be pain free but may produce gentle pulling sensations as contractile and noncontractile tissues are stretched.
7. When attempting to improve flexibility, athletes must enhance collagen's plasticity component through prolonged stretching.
8. The tissue to be stretched should be warm before stretching to maximize stretching efforts. This can be accomplished by gentle warm-up activities or by applying therapeutic heating modalities.
9. Stretching must be done to the point of an uncomfortable pulling sensation and then held there for 6 to 30 seconds. Overstretching is harmful and is characterized by involuntary muscle quivering, a breakdown in proper form, or poststretching pain.
10. You can be of particular assistance by spotting improper form in the athlete's stretching program.

Chapter 10
Exercises to Increase Muscle Strength

This chapter provides guidelines and specific tasks that you can use to ensure that your athletes' muscles get adequate, sport-specific strengthening.

Muscle provides for active joint movement and serves as a dynamic backup to joint stability. When muscle strength is inadequate, the joint is more susceptible to injury. Another contributing factor to some sport injuries is inadequate muscle strength.

Muscle is injured when muscle strength is not sufficient to meet the demands of a particular sport. Another factor in acute muscle injury is an inappropriate agonist-to-antagonist muscle strength ratio.

It is therefore no surprise that when efforts to strengthen muscle following sport injury fail, the most common reasons are that the strengthening program was inadequate in terms of addressing the demands of sport and it was not specific to the structures involved.

BENEFITS OF STRENGTHENING

As muscle becomes stronger, it is able to generate greater work. Muscle strengthening, whether done with weights, conditioning drills, or another form of external resistance, benefits other tissues as well. Strengthening exercises not only create strong muscles but also strengthen tendons, bones, and ligaments.

Efforts to increase strength in sport-specific patterns (jumping, bounding, throwing) help to make muscles functionally strong. Repetition of these patterns also helps to make movement more automatic, more efficient, and better coordinated. Thus, proper strengthening programs serve to improve performance and help decrease certain injuries. However, muscle strength alone does not guarantee that the joints those particular muscles surround will not be injured. Adequate ROM and, yes, good fortune are also necessary for athletes to participate free from injury.

I limit my discussion of strengthening to its role in the rehabilitation process. Strength training can be accomplished in a number of innovative ways. Most of the exercises described in this chapter can be easily applied in a school's weight room, a local health club, or an athlete's home or dorm room. And many of the activities can be used in injury prevention programs that concentrate on muscles vital to participation in a given sport.

Because of the intricacies of sport rehabilitation, general program development should be left to a trained medical specialist. And a certified strength-training coach can be very valuable for ensuring that the program is properly implemented once it is developed.

TYPES OF MUSCLE CONTRACTIONS

Before you can implement a specific strengthening program, you must understand how muscles work. An in-depth discussion of the sliding-filament hypothesis, the neurophysiology of muscle contraction and relaxation, and other principles are well beyond the scope of this book. Rather, my discussion of muscle activity concentrates on the basic contractions:

- concentric,
- eccentric, and
- isometric.

Concentric (Shortening) Contraction

When we think of typical muscle contraction, we usually envision *concentric* contraction. This is a shortening contraction of the muscle in which the origin and the insertion of the muscle come closer together.

An example of concentric (positive) muscle work is seated knee extension. The athlete sits on a weight bench with the knee flexed at a comfortable resting position. As the athlete extends the knee, muscle filaments slide and the muscle shortens, pulling the insertion of the quadriceps on the tibia closer to the muscle's origin along the upper femur and pelvis.

Vital to smooth muscular contraction is a finely tuned interaction between agonist and antagonist. A complex neurophysiological principle called *reciprocal innervation* allows for controlled relaxation of the antagonist as the agonist produces work. In knee extension, the quadriceps shorten to extend the knee, and the hamstrings relax sufficiently to allow the knee to straighten.

Eccentric (Lengthening) Contraction

An *eccentric* (negative) contraction is a lengthening contraction of the muscle in which muscle fibers elongate under tension to allow the distance between the origin and the insertion of the muscle to become greater.

Referring back to the knee extension example, as the athlete slowly lowers the leg from a fully extended position to a flexed starting position, the quadriceps generate tension as the muscle fibers elongate.

Isometric Contraction

In an *isometric* contraction, muscle force is generated, but the joint on which the muscles act does not move. Thus, there is no change in the length of the muscle: The muscle's origin and insertion move neither closer to nor further from each other.

Once again, knee extension provides a good example. This time the athlete places the foot under an 800-pound barbell and is asked to extend the knee. The athlete cannot overcome the resistance, but the quadriceps are working even though there is no joint motion.

Isometrics can also be performed when the external resistance is applied by the agonist. In this case, the athlete extends the knee with no weighted resistance to a given point in the motion. The athlete is then asked to hold the leg at this point. If the knee is kept at that angle with the quadriceps and hamstrings working, this isometric co-contraction generates force without subsequent joint motion.

Muscle Contractions With Resistance

To build on our basics, shortening and lengthening contractions can be classified as isotonic and isokinetic.

Isotonic Muscular Work

Isotonic refers to constant resistance applied to a muscle throughout a given ROM. Let's use the knee extension example again. If we placed a 30-pound weight around the athlete's ankle and asked the athlete to extend the knee, he or she would be performing isotonic exercise. The 30-pound resistance remains constant through the full ROM.

Isotonics are commonly used to strengthen muscle. Ankle weights, barbells, Universal and Nautilus equipment, and weighted bats and balls are all used in isotonic exercise. Strength gains are made by overloading the muscle to make it work progressively harder. The harder the muscle works, the stronger the muscle becomes. By placing additional stress on the muscle, it must work harder to overcome that stress. The additional stress produces additional muscle strength. This *overload principle* is at the heart of effective muscle strengthening.

Muscle shortening occurs as muscle filaments slide past one another while maintaining contact to generate force. In every joint's ROM is a point (usually in the midrange of a given motion) at which a maximum number of muscle filaments are in contact with one another and at which the muscle is able to generate its maximum force.

For example, as knee extension begins with the knee bent, the quadriceps are in a lengthened state. As the knee straightens, the filaments slide by one another to a point at which the maximum number of quadriceps filaments are in contact with one another. As further extension occurs, the filaments slide past one another as the quadriceps become fully shortened at full extension. Therefore, to complete full knee extension, the quadriceps must generate enough force at their weakest point to overcome the weight of the lower leg plus the weight of the resistance. In knee extension it is usually most difficult for the quadriceps to generate force as the knee approaches full extension. Little difficulty in lifting a weight is encountered in the midrange of knee extension. However, as the knee straightens, more effort is required to move the weight. Isotonics, therefore, are a true assessment only of the muscle's strength through the full ROM at the muscle's weakest point in the ROM.

Isokinetic Muscular Work

Isokinetic refers to resistance applied at a constant speed throughout the ROM. Once the desired speed of motion is attained, resistance applied to the muscle is constant, so the joint cannot move at a speed greater than the preset velocity of motion.

Formal testing of muscle strength at sports medicine clinics is often done isokinetically. Knee extension is routinely tested at 60° per second in tests of the quadriceps. That is, the velocity, or speed of motion, is set so that the knee moves no greater than 60° of extension per second. Once the athlete is able to move the joint at 60° per second, the quadriceps meet the resistance of the machine, which remains at the constant speed and allows the quadriceps to work as hard as possible through the full ROM. The athlete generates force (measured in foot pounds of torque) at the maximum capability as long as effort is maximal and the speed of movement constant. In this way, a true assessment is made of muscle strength throughout the full ROM rather than the muscle's strength at its weakest point in the ROM (isotonics).

The sophistication of isokinetic strengthening and strength-testing apparatus has increased dramatically. Cybex, Kin-Com, Biodex,

and Lido are but a few of the isokinetic units frequently used today. Another form of isokinetics is hydraulic resisted strengthening. In these units, hydraulic resistance allows motion to be performed at a speed no greater than what the unit is preset to allow. Once the resistance is met at the preset speed, resistance remains constant at a fixed speed of movement. Higher settings require that more force be exerted to meet the increased resistance at the same speed.

Comparisons of Muscle Contractions

With all the types of muscle contractions and the various ways to stress muscle, it can be difficult to decide which method to use. Each method as it relates to the rehabilitation process has advantages and disadvantages.

Concentric Versus Eccentric Versus Isometric

Concentric muscle contraction is an effective means of stressing muscle tissue and can easily be performed with a variety of readily available equipment. Eccentric muscle contractions isolate stresses on the muscle tendon more effectively than does concentric work. Muscles are also able to generate greater forces eccentrically. However, eccentric contractions have been shown to increase postexercise delayed muscle soreness.

Isometrics are joint-angle specific. That is, gains in strength made isometrically occur only in a small ROM corresponding to the angle of motion in which the isometrics are performed. Because no joint motion occurs with isometrics, these exercises can be performed with little stress on or damage to joint structures.

Isotonics Versus Isokinetics

The availability of isotonic exercise apparatus is certainly greater than that of isokinetic equipment. Major reasons for this include its relative ease of use and its low cost.

Isokinetic exercise equipment is advantageous in that it can be set up to isolate muscle groups and provide resistance through the full ROM.

ASSESSING MUSCLE STRENGTH

Several methods of muscle strength measurement are possible, ranging from the inexpensive and unsophisticated to the expensive and elaborate.

Manual Muscle Tests

Rehabilitation specialists isolate a given muscle group, then apply manual resistance to the body part being tested. The examiner then determines the amount of resistance tolerated by the athlete and assigns an appropriate grade to the muscle. Although the grades and the criteria are standardized, a degree of subjectivity is still involved on the examiner's part.

More objective measures of strength include the cable tensiometer, the hand-held dynamometer, and the isokinetic dynamometer.

Cable Tensiometer

The tensiometer, particularly useful in early studies of muscle strength, provides an accurate assessment of strength. The body part to be tested exerts a pulling force on a cable that is attached to the body part. A corresponding measurement is read from a force gauge that is attached to the opposite end of the cable. Although the tensiometer is accurate it is specific only to the point in the ROM to which stress is applied.

Hand-Held Dynamometer

This device can be applied to two types of strength assessment. The true hand-held dynamometer measures grip strength. It is held by the person being evaluated and is squeezed as hard as possible. A reading of the force exerted is taken from the dynamometer's gauge.

Another type of dynamometer is one that the examiner, not the subject, holds. The body part to be assessed is isolated as in the manual muscle test. The muscles being tested contract against resistance applied by the dynamometer, and the generated value of force is read from the gauge. Thus, this assessment differs from the manual muscle test, but only because an objective number, not a subjective examiner's grade, is used to assess function.

Isokinetic Dynamometer

By far, isokinetic dynamometers are the most frequently used objective methods to measure muscle strength. Today's isokinetic units are versatile in that they can evaluate every major joint in the body (except the fingers and toes). Such units are also technologically sophisticated, as isokinetic speeds can be adjusted from 1° per second to over 400° per second.

Both concentric and eccentric strength can be assessed on most machines. Computer-assisted data analysis yields a tremendous amount of information regarding the specific muscle group tested. These highly accurate machines are now commonplace in most sports medicine centers.

Strength can be assessed accurately through the desired ROM rather than at only one point in the range. The only drawback to these units is their cost, as most are priced between $30,000 and $50,000.

INDICATORS OF INSUFFICIENT MUSCLE STRENGTH

Muscle strength is insufficient to perform a task if

- the athlete cannot complete the exercise through the desired ROM,
- the athlete cannot complete the desired number of sets or repetitions, or
- involuntary muscle shaking or an inability to control movement occurs during the task.

If any of these signs are present, stress applied to the muscle must be temporarily decreased by

- decreasing the weight the athlete is attempting to lift or
- decreasing the number of repetitions or sets performed.

ELEMENTS OF STRENGTH-CONDITIONING SESSIONS

As is the case with flexibility and ROM exercises, opinions differ regarding strengthening exercise form, duration, frequency, recovery time, and progression. Remember, we are considering strengthening work specific to rehabilitation, not off-season weight training or bodybuilding conducted as part of in-season practices.

Form

Proper form is important when performing strengthening exercises. The muscle to be strengthened must be isolated. If the number of repetitions or the amount of resistance is excessive, stronger or uninvolved muscles will be used instead.

Another common way that proper form breaks down is when the involved muscle fatigues and the athlete attempts to use momentum to compensate for the fatigue. Failure to complete a given exercise through the full ROM is another way that proper exercise form breaks down. You should observe your athletes closely when they perform strengthening activities, checking for both improper form and the use of momentum.

Duration

In the acute phase, exercise (if pain-free) can be performed three or four times a day. Active exercise in the acute phase with gravity either eliminated or assisting motion helps to maintain muscle tone. Three sets of 15 to 20 repetitions are usually sufficient to encourage fluid movement, nourish articular cartilage, and maintain pain-free ROM.

If muscle has atrophied in the subacute phase and into the chronic phase, more repetitions with lower weight may prove beneficial. Red muscle fibers are the first to atrophy after immobilization. Red fibers are responsible for the slow-twitch muscle activity usually involved in endurance work. Therefore, when atrophy is present, assume that there is some

red-fiber involvement. To stimulate these slow-twitch muscle fibers, have the athlete perform three or four sets of high-repetition (30 to 40) exercises.

Frequency (Recovery Time)

More time for recovery should be allowed during the acute phase than during the subacute and chronic phases. This additional recovery time will help the athlete determine how he or she is tolerating a given exercise. If repetitions are not graduated and recovery time is insufficient, the athlete may have an increase in swelling, pain, or both. Recovery time of 3 to 5 minutes between sets is adequate.

Less recovery time is necessary during the subacute and chronic phases. Tests have shown that a given muscle will usually recover sufficiently to perform a subsequent set of exercise at an appropriate level after about 1-1/2 minutes. Athletes should exercise a few times per day during the acute phase and then once per day in the subacute phase. Maintenance and strength-building work can be performed every other day once symmetry is gained with the opposite side.

WARNING SIGNALS OF OVERSTRESSING MUSCLES

Signs that a muscle is being overstressed are

- muscle pain while performing a given task,
- failure of a muscle to recover after adequate rest between sets or workouts, and
- failure to increase the amount of weight lifted or the number of repetitions performed.

Progression of Strengthening Exercises

Because postinjury muscle tissue is usually weakened, it is vital to be able to test muscle strength to determine a baseline point from which subsequent progress can be measured. Normal muscle testing grades were developed for this purpose. A trained examiner needs to perform the testing to accurately isolate and grade muscle function. Muscle test grades range from 0 through 5 or from "zero" through "normal" (see Table 10.1). Rarely are the muscle grades of "zero" and "trace" seen in sport rehabilitation. However, as a result of pain, swelling, muscle trauma, or other reasons, poor muscle grades are commonly seen in acute athletic injury.

Table 10.1
Muscle Grades

Grade	Rating (out of 5)	Joint motion description
Normal	5	Full AROM against gravity; able to tolerate maximum manual resistance applied to the muscle
Good	4	Same as normal grade but able to tolerate only submaximal resistance
Fair	3	Full AROM against gravity
Poor	2	Able to complete full AROM in a position with gravity eliminated
Trace	1	Muscle contracts but produces no joint motion
Zero	0	No muscle contraction observed or felt

Weakness accompanied by pain can be helpful in implicating muscle involvement after injury. Weakness without pain, however, may signal more severe involvement, ranging from peripheral nerve damage to complete tendon rupture to nonorthopedic pathology. When muscle strength is poor, strengthening efforts should include activities that eliminate the effect of gravity and allow the muscles to move a given joint through the available ROM. The weight of the involved body part in a gravity-eliminated position usually provides enough resistance during this phase. Pain-free isometrics may also be beneficial in this stage.

As muscle function improves and strength increases, the athlete can begin moving the body part against gravity (a muscle grade of "fair"). Assistance may be needed at the ends

of ROMs as muscle strength in the shortened position may be insufficient to complete movement through the full range. Remember, muscle is able to generate more force eccentrically, so eccentric strengthening work at the ends of ROMs is often helpful for muscles with a "fair" strength grade.

Once the involved joint can complete full ROM against gravity, outside resistance may be applied in addition to the weight of the body part against gravity ("good" or "normal" muscle grades). Manual resistance and isotonic and isokinetic concentric and eccentric work may now be performed. Specific strengthening exercises and progressions for given joints as they relate to common sport injuries are discussed later in this chapter.

ADJUNCTIVE MEANS TO PROMOTE STRENGTHENING

Two common therapeutic muscle-strengthening modalities that have not been discussed are surface electromyographic biofeedback and functional electrical stimulation.

Electromyographic Biofeedback

Muscles contract by way of electrical impulses propagated along the paths of motor nerves. Muscle contraction has an inherent electrical activity that can be recorded by a technique called *electromyography* (EMG). Needles, or electrodes, are placed in the muscle or on the skin (surface EMG). The electrical output of the muscle is picked up by the electrodes and fed into a biofeedback unit. Baseline audio or visual signals projected on a monitor are generated by the muscle. When the muscle contracts, the audio signal intensifies or the visual recording of the muscle's response shows a corresponding deflection on the monitor. By keying in to the audio or visual feedback mechanism, the athlete can increase muscle response voluntarily.

Functional Electrical Stimulation

After prolonged joint immobilization or in cases of acute injury in which pain or swelling prevents selective muscle function, *func-*

tional electrical stimulation (FES) can assist the rehabilitation process. The unit produces an electrical current with a wavelength and pulse that stimulate skeletal muscle effectively. Larger units are electrically operated, and the small, portable units are battery operated. Electrodes from the unit are attached to the skin over the muscle to be stimulated, and a current is generated to produce a muscle contraction.

Point stimulation at a motor point (where a motor nerve enters a muscle) by a hand-held stimulator is especially useful for small muscles. Studies have shown that electrical stimulation helps to increase muscle strength when done in conjunction with simultaneous muscle contraction. The contraindications and precautions for functional electrical stimulation are the same as those for the electrotherapeutic modalities discussed in chapter 6.

EXERCISES TO INCREASE MUSCLE STRENGTH

The therapeutic strengthening exercises prescribed for athletes will vary depending on their state of rehabilitation. Many of these exercises can also be implemented in preseason conditioning and in-season maintenance programs in an effort to prevent injury.

General Guidelines for a Successful Strengthening Program

1. Begin with gentle warm-up activities to elevate muscle temperature, then follow these with static stretching of the involved muscle group or body part.
2. In the acute phase, perform active, pain-free midrange ROM work in a gravity-assisted or gravity-eliminated position. If AROM is painful, even in a limited range, the athlete should instead perform submaximal isometrics in the pain-free range.
3. Subacute-phase resistance can be increased in the midrange and then decreased at the ends of motion until work is pain free and symmetry achieved with the uninvolved side.
4. Resistance should be deemphasized until the involved body part can complete full AROM against gravity.
5. The athlete should maintain high repetitions (three sets of 30 reps) in the acute and subacute phases with little resistance. Once the high reps are tolerated, the athlete should add weighted resistance.
6. When repetitions are completed through the full ROM with no sensation of muscle fatigue, the athletes should add 1 to 2 pounds for the upper extremities and 3 to 5 pounds for the lower extremities.
7. When utilizing weight machines designed to work either both arms or both legs, modify the technique to isolate the athlete's involved side for three sets of 30 reps and the noninjured side for three sets of 10 to 15 reps.
8. Strengthening work should follow warm-ups, stretches, and any sport-related activity. For example, when the athlete is able to bicycle, swim, or run for cardiovascular conditioning but is not able to practice or compete, strengthening should follow the aerobic exercise. And, when the athlete begins functional progression drills or modified or actual sport participation, strengthening activities should follow these sport-related activities.
9. After strengthening work, stretching should be performed to maintain flexibility and minimize postexercise muscle soreness.
10. Ice should be applied to the involved area after activity, especially if it is painful or swollen.

The guidelines on the previous page will help you identify strength deficiencies and monitor your athletes' strengthening progress through the rehabilitation program.

Acute-Phase Strengthening Exercises

Strengthening activities of all body regions should be performed with caution. And absolutely no vigorous strengthening work should be performed acutely until an accurate diagnosis has been made.

Neck (Cervical Spine)

After acute injury to neck muscles or ligamentous structures, rest is required to allow the injury to resolve. This rest may range from a few days of sitting out of activity to being immobilized in a neck brace.

When acute symptoms subside, athletes can perform gentle, pain-free AROM, including forward flexion (chin to chest), lateral flexion (ear to shoulder), and rotation (looking over either shoulder). Extension may need to be avoided in the acute phase. Following mild injuries, athletes may be able to perform pain-free midrange submaximal isometric contractions. To do so, the athlete places his or her hand on the forehead and gently applies force into the hand with the head. Similar isometric resistance can be applied at each side of the head (for lateral flexion and rotation) and at the back of the head (for extension).

Adequate strength of the neck muscles is an absolute prerequisite for contact sports because it helps dissipate both direct forces to the delicate cervical spine and indirect forces to the spinal cord and the brain. Neck strength is even more vital for athletes who might be predisposed to potential head and neck injuries (long-necked individuals).

Shoulder and Shoulder Girdle

Traumatic acute athletic injuries involving the shoulder (glenohumeral) joint include subluxations, dislocations, and contusions. Fractures and other serious injuries are less common.

After acute injury, the shoulder is often immobilized by a sling or a sling and swath. When pain has sufficiently subsided, gentle, pain-free isometrics may be performed, even with the arm in the sling. In-sling isometric contractions can be performed by pushing the lower arm into the stomach or pushing the arm away from the stomach as the opposite hand provides resistance. When allowed, unresisted elbow flexion and extension can be performed. And, if pain free, athletes may perform unresisted shoulder shrugs or may even squeeze the shoulder blades together. However, particularly with acromioclavicular joint involvement, such activities may be too painful.

Elbow, Wrist, and Hand

Acute conditions of the elbow, wrist, and hand occur frequently in sport. Fractures of these body parts, dislocations of the elbow, and tendon injuries of the hand all warrant special evaluation.

After acute injury to the elbow, the involved arm is often placed in a sling or other form of immobilization. If pain free, the immobilized parts may be removed from protection and moved through AROM. Encourage the athlete to move the shoulders and all healthy joints through pain-free AROM two or three times a day.

Lower Back (Lumbar Spine)

Lower back injuries range from the serious to the minor. Serious injury to the back can arise acutely, such as a fracture that results in paraplegia. Minor acute injuries involving the muscles and ligaments of the lumbar region can often be prevented from becoming chronic through exercise.

Strengthening exercises are usually deemphasized in acute lower back injury, as even gentle strengthening efforts often result in increased muscle spasm and pain. In fact, just getting into a prone position to perform strengthening exercises may increase paravertebral spasm. Therefore, rest is usually prescribed for 1 or 2 days following injury to the lower back. However, gentle motion can be allowed if the athlete experiences no pain.

Hip, Groin, and Pelvis

The hip joint is perhaps the most stable joint of the body. But acute muscle strains involving the hip flexors and adductors occur frequently.

To strengthen the hip joint effectively, the athlete must move the joint against gravity. However, because the weight of the entire leg must be moved, even simple gravity-resisted exercise may prove too strenuous in the acute phase. In these cases, exercise should be performed in the pain-free range with gravity eliminated. The athlete can perform hip flexion and extension while lying on the uninvolved side. Abduction and adduction, as well as internal and external rotation, can also be performed by the athlete lying on the back.

Midrange isometrics against manual resistance or against resistance offered by the other leg may also be beneficial in the acute phase. If the hip flexor is involved, the athlete can sit with the knee bent and a hand resting on the knee of the injured leg. Keeping the hand in this position, the athlete can try to lift the leg against the resistance of the hand. If an adductor is involved, isometrics can be performed by placing a pillow, a volleyball, or both of the athlete's fists between the knees. Keeping the knees straight, the athlete squeezes the legs together against the object placed between the knees. Remember, if a gravity-resisted motion is painful, the athlete should avoid it. And all pain-free motion at the hip should be encouraged.

Knee

Tremendous strides have been made in the last 10 years in understanding knee injuries, surgical procedures of the knee, and post- and nonoperative rehabilitation techniques. Some rehabilitation procedures, especially improperly designed strengthening programs, have now been shown to be ineffective and sometimes detrimental. Thus proper knee care is absolutely essential for the success of a sport rehabilitation program, as the knee is the most frequently injured joint in sport.

After acute knee injury, quadriceps function may decrease within hours. When indicated, isometrics of the quadriceps can be instituted as tolerated and eventually increased to 300 to 400 8-second contractions per day. Isometrics of the quadriceps, called *quad sets*, should be performed with the knee bent slightly and must be pain free.

Although hamstring function does not decrease as greatly as quadriceps function after surgery or acute knee injury, hamstring-

strengthening isometrics are important, especially after anterior cruciate injury. Hamstring isometrics are performed with the athlete lying on the back and bending the knee to about 90°. Keeping the knee bent at this angle, the athlete tries to push the heel of the involved leg into the surface he or she is lying on.

Calf, Ankle, and Foot

Acute ankle sprains are common in sport. In fact, in some sports, ankle injuries (usually sprains) are more frequent than knee injuries. The ankle, calf, and foot also suffer acute tendon strains and avulsions, calf muscle tears, Achilles tendon ruptures, and other soft-tissue problems.

Pain-free AROM not only assists in maintaining muscle strength after acute injury but, when combined with elevation, also helps decrease swelling. Midrange pain-free isometrics or manual resisted motion can also be performed as the athlete applies resistance with the hands. The foot can be pulled back toward the lower leg or pushed down and away from the lower leg against the resistance provided by the hand. Also, the foot can be turned in toward the opposite foot or turned away from the opposite leg. Remember, especially after ankle sprain, the motion that was responsible for initially injuring the ankle should be avoided.

Subacute-Phase Strengthening Exercises

During the subacute phase, you should emphasize graduated strengthening work through the full ROM. Movements should be kept pain free, initial resistance applied to the involved structure should be light, and repetitions should be high.

Neck

As the ROM of the neck returns to normal, strengthening activities should be progressed. Submaximal isometrics can be performed at multiple points in the range of flexion, extension, lateral flexion, and rotation, with each contraction lasting 5 to 8 seconds. Once these submaximal isometrics are tolerated, maximal isometric contractions may be attempted.

When the neck has full, pain-free AROM and can generate maximal isometric force, more resistance can be added. Football players often perform exercises with partners in which one player alternately applies manual resistance to each side of a partner's head. Resistance can increase as far as the athlete can tolerate. Spring-loaded resistance is available on some forms of strengthening equipment (Universal), whereas others offer an individual station for weight-resisted neck strengthening. Head harnesses, in which weights are added to the end of the harness, can also be used.

Shoulder and Shoulder Girdle

Active ROM at the shoulder should progress gradually over shoulder height. As discomfort allows, strengthening work may be added above shoulder height gradually. When unresisted overhead motion is pain free, the athlete may begin resisted work with weights or surgical tubing.

Shoulder dislocation usually produces weak spots in the front part of the shoulder capsule. Maximal stress is placed on the capsule after dislocation when the shoulder is abducted to about 90° and then externally rotated (see Figure 10.1). Vigorous strengthening (resistance set to achieve muscle fatigue at the end of the workout) of the middle and anterior deltoids and of the shoulder's internal rotators is important after dislocation.

A particularly effective way to strengthen the internal rotators of the shoulder is to apply resistance with surgical tubing (see Figure 10.2). Muscles of the rotator cuff also need to be strengthened by external rotation, but exercises for this purpose should not be done with the shoulder abducted.

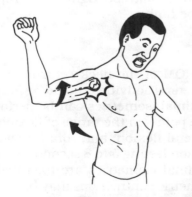

Figure 10.1. Position of maximum vulnerability after anterior shoulder dislocation.

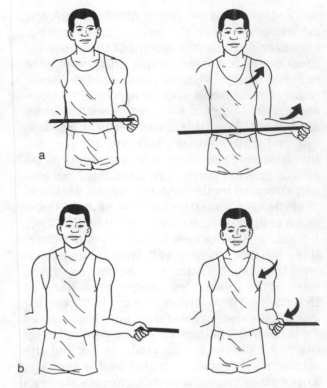

Figure 10.2. Resistance strengthening exercises for the external and internal rotators of the shoulder using surgical tubing: a, external shoulder rotation; b, internal shoulder rotation.

Elbow, Wrist, and Hand

Submaximal to maximal grip activities help to maintain forearm muscle tone and decrease swelling. Wrist curls (flexion) and reverse curls (extension) done with dumbbells, barbells, or wrist rollers, can increase strength of the wrists and forearms. When only one arm is involved, dumbbells or other forms of one-sided resisted work may be most beneficial. Encourage the athlete to strengthen both sides of the arm, but one side at a time.

Wrist pronation and supination can be difficult to strengthen specifically. Manual resisted exercise using the opposite, noninvolved side may help. Or, a hammer offers a practical and efficient method of resistance. When the muscles are weak, the athlete should grip the hammer close to its head. As the athlete's strength increases, the grip can be moved down the handle. A grip farther from the hammer's head places more resistance on the athlete's wrist, making efforts more difficult.

Lower Back

For the paravertebrals, the best way to start is in the prone position. With the arms straight overhead, the athlete lifts the left arm and right leg off the floor or treatment table approximately 4 to 6 inches. After holding the position for 5 seconds, the athlete lowers the arm and leg and repeats the exercise with the right arm and left leg. When this is tolerated well, the athlete places the arms down at the side and, with the legs and hips flat on the floor or treatment table, raises the trunk 6 to 8 inches off the surface he or she is lying on. Once this is tolerated well, the arms are then placed back with the hands resting on top of the head. Only after this is easy for the athlete to perform should weight machines designed for the back be used or should exercises begin in which the athlete actively extends the entire upper half of the body off the edge of the treatment table.

During the subacute phase, athletes with lower back injury should also strengthen the gluteus maximus, latissimus dorsi, and abdominals.

Hip, Groin, and Pelvis

When the hip joint can be moved through the full ROM against gravity, resistance may be added. For example, hip flexion during straight-leg raises can be stressed with ankle weights or a weight boot adding resistance. Straight-leg raises should be performed with the opposite leg flexed at the hip and knee to minimize stress placed on the lower back (see Figure 10.3).

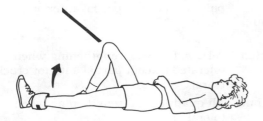

Figure 10.3. Straight-leg raises for hip flexor strengthening.

One-joint hip flexors (iliopsoas), isolated with exaggerated hip flexion in the standing position (marching), can be resisted with weights around the thigh or the ankle. Resistance with surgical tubing can be added in this position or while the athlete is on the hands and knees performing a knee-to-chest motion (see Figure 10.4).

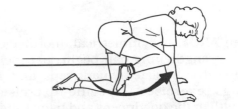

Figure 10.4. Resistance strengthening exercise for hip flexors using surgical tubing.

Prone hip extension with the knee extended stresses all the hip extensors, including the hamstrings. Isolation of the gluteus maximus is achieved by hip extension with the knee flexed to 90°. Gravity-resisted adduction with weights or adduction resisted with tubing can also be employed (see Figure 10.5).

When stressing hip abduction to isolate the gluteus medius, the athlete's hip must be in a slightly extended position. Side leg lifts to strengthen the hip abductors are commonly assisted by the quadriceps when the hip is not extended slightly. Again, weight- or tubing-resisted exercises are effective for strengthening. Resistance applied to strengthen hip rotators is best done in a seated position. Manual resistance applied at the lower leg, ankle weights, tubing, or Theraband resistance applied just above the ankle is also sufficient.

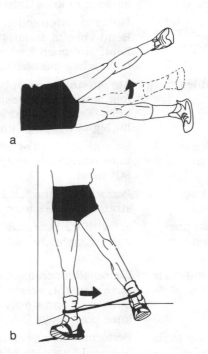

Figure 10.5. Strengthening exercises for hip adductors: a, gravity-resisted side leg lifts; b, resisted standing adduction using surgical tubing.

Knee

When AROM is symmetrical, more vigorous knee strengthening can begin that includes progressive, resisted quadriceps and hamstrings exercises. Specific exercises to strengthen the quadriceps and hamstrings are described in Table 10.2.

In addition to these exercises, isotonics, multiple-angle isometrics, and isokinetics can be used. Body weight resistance drills such as step-ups can also be added as tolerated. Refer to Table 10.2 if you are concerned whether certain knee exercises are indicated or contra-indicated for a given injury.

Calf, Ankle, and Foot

More vigorous strengthening can begin once nonresisted, full AROM is painfree. Manual resisted exercise, surgical tubing or Thera-band resistance, and weight resistance are all effective strengthening methods.

For common inversion ankle sprains, exercises to strengthen the dorsiflexors and evertors should be used (see Figure 10.6).

Subacute-phase calf strains or contusions also require dorsiflexor, evertor, and invertor strengthening in addition to exercises of the calf muscles themselves. The athlete should perform toe raises in the standing position using both the involved and the uninvolved leg. Bearing weight on both sides, the athlete should lift the heels up while standing on the toes of both feet. This exercise should first be performed on a flat surface. As the athlete is able to bear more weight on the affected side, the toe raises should stress the involved side only. And, when the athlete is able to do single-leg (affected side) toe raises on a flat surface, he or she can then attempt toe raises on both sides from an incline. In this case, the

Table 10.2
Quadriceps and Hamstring Strengthening Exercises

Exercises	Descriptions	Indications
Quadriceps set	Isometric contraction of quadriceps: With knee straight, tighten quadriceps as back of knee flattens out.	Acute phase of all knee injuries when pain free (except partial anterior cruciate tears)
Hamstring set	Isometric contraction of hamstrings: Bend knee to about 45°, keep knee bent, and push heel of involved leg back while maintaining 45° bend.	Acute anterior cruciate tears and hamstring injuries
Straight-leg raise	Lie flat and bend opposite knee so that foot is flat and opposite the involved knee. Keep involved knee straight and lift leg to height of uninvolved leg.	Acute phase of all knee injuries when pain free (except partial anterior cruciate tears)
Full knee extension	Sit with leg bent at 90° angle. Straighten knee completely and slowly return to 90° bend.	All quadriceps strengthening when tolerated (except partial anterior cruciate tears)
Partial knee extension	Perform like the full knee extension, but straighten knee from 90° to only 40°.	All quadriceps strengthening when tolerated
Terminal knee extension	Sit with leg bent at 30° angle. Straighten knee completely and slowly return to 30° bend.	When emphasizing vastus medialis strengthening (patellar subluxation and dislocation)
Hamstring curls (neutral)	Lie on stomach (prone) and start with knee straight, slowly bend knee (heel to buttocks), and slowly return to straight-knee position.	All anterior cruciate ligament tears and hamstring injuries.
Hamstring curls (externally rotated)	Performed like neutral hamstring curls, but turn lower leg so that foot and toes point out, away from opposite foot.	Anterior cruciate tears with rotatory instability (anterolateral)

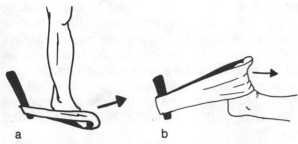

Figure 10.6. Theraband strengthening exercises for the ankle: a, evertors; b, dorsiflexors.

athlete stands with the balls of the feet resting on a surface, then lowers the heels to 3 to 4 inches below the edge of the surface. These toe raises should be performed with both legs before the athlete uses only the involved leg. Progression exercises for this activity include performing toe raises while wearing a weighted backpack, holding a dumbbell in each hand, or standing over the benchpress station on a Universal machine and grasping the handles.

Chronic-Phase Strengthening Exercises

Inadequate strength is a common component of chronic sport injury. As we saw, pain resulting from injury produces weak muscles that, if not addressed with specific strengthening exercises, remain weak and susceptible to re-injury. So let's look at some strengthening exercises that may help decrease the likelihood of an injury becoming chronic.

Neck

Recurrent neck strains and sprains and brachial plexus stretches (burners and stingers) must be thoroughly evaluated for a predisposing skeletal abnormality. Once this examination is completed, exercises that strengthen the neck muscles may provide dynamic support to the injured area. Because brachial plexus stretches occur with lateral flexion of the neck to one side with simultaneous depression of the shoulder on the opposite side, strengthening of the sternocleidomastoids, levator scapulae, and upper trapezius is essential.

The sternocleidomastoid on the right side is isolated by looking up and back over the left shoulder. No machine can adequately strengthen this muscle, so manual resistance is the best way to selectively strengthen it. As the sternocleidomastoid also is a primary neck flexor, flexion exercises are also effective ways to strengthen it. Isotonic machines are designed for such exercises, and resistance can be offered by a stack of weights or a spring.

A shoulder shrug (i.e., bringing the shoulder blades to the ears) is an appropriate strengthening exercise that recruits the upper trapezius and levator scapulae. Shrugs can be effectively resisted by using the bench-press station of the Universal, by using dumbbells or a barbell, or by standing on a loop of surgical tubing.

Shoulder and Shoulder Girdle

Shoulder dislocation can become a chronic problem, especially if the athlete is young when the first dislocation occurs. Perhaps more common is recurrent shoulder subluxation. Strengthening the anterior and middle deltoid, rotator cuff, and pectoralis major muscles is important.

The anterior deltoid and pectoralis groups can be effectively strengthened with horizontal adduction exercises, which involve pulling the arm over and across the chest. Nautilus butterfly stations work well for this. However, when doing butterfly-type motions, the athlete should not let the upper arm extend backward past a position that is even with the shoulder.

Surgical tubing work that stresses internal rotation will strengthen the pectorals and parts of the rotator cuff. External rotation work with tubing will work the remaining portions of the cuff muscles.

Another chronic overuse injury of the shoulder is impingement syndrome. Strengthening exercises help to manage this problem. As described in chapter 4, impingement syndrome is caused by the supraspinatus or the biceps tendon (or both) being pinched between the humerus and the coracoacromial ligament. Strengthening exercises that depress the humeral head and provide more room for the tendons are beneficial. The primary muscle group serving this function is the rotator cuff. Therefore, internal and external rotation exercises are essential.

Because the supraspinatus muscle is the primary structure pinched, this muscle must be strengthened so it can more effectively assist in depressing the humeral head. The supraspinatus can be isolated by the empty-can exercise (see Figure 10.7). A strong supraspinatus assists in lowering the humerus in the glenoid cavity. Scapular rotators should be strengthened as well to raise the roof of the coracoacromial ligament complex.

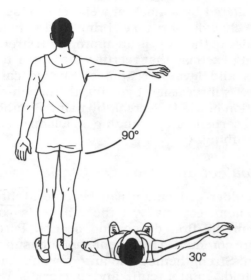

Figure 10.7. Empty-can exercise to isolate the supraspinatus muscle.

Impingement syndrome can be managed through serratus anterior strengthening exercises that allow more efficient upward scapular rotation. The serratus anterior muscle can be strengthened by wall push-ups and by terminal motions of bench pressing, in which the weight is held with the elbows locked and completely extended and then pushed toward the ceiling. Accessory muscles for scapular stability can be strengthened by upright rowing.

Elbow, Wrist, and Hand

Two common and sometimes chronic elbow problems are medial elbow overload and lateral epicondylitis (tennis elbow). Strengthening is an important part of the total treatment plan for these two challenging conditions.

In medial overload, the primary muscle groups to strengthen are those of the medial forearm flexor and pronators. Thus, the athlete should first perform resisted wrist flexion with the elbow bent to approximately 90° and then work into more elbow extension. Barbells, dumbbells, and surgical tubing are good methods to strengthen the wrist flexors. Pronation strengthening with isolated pronation

at 90° of elbow flexion and in combination with simultaneous wrist and elbow flexion should be done to provide dynamic stability for the area. As previously noted, a hammer is an excellent device to strengthen the pronators. Grasp-strengthening exercises that use spring-loaded resistance devices or squeezing a tennis ball are also effective for medial overload.

Tennis elbow is one of the most challenging conditions to rehabilitate. Strengthening efforts should emphasize wrist extensors, flexors, pronators, and supinators. Particularly beneficial is strengthening the wrist extensors through negative or lengthening contractions. Eccentric (negative) contractions place stress on the tendinous structures of the muscle-tendon unit. Negatives can be isolated simply by letting the wrist lower slowly to a resting flexed position after completing a reverse wrist curl.

Progressing to faster speeds of lengthening contractions puts more stress on the involved area. Proper performance and gradual advancement of an eccentric loading program are significant parts of the rehabilitation program for tennis elbow. The athlete with this condition should perform three sets of 10 repetitions, starting at a slow speed and gradually advancing to faster speeds. A medically trained professional should be consulted for specific instruction on form and for general troubleshooting.

Lower Back

Chronic lower back pain is another challenging clinical condition. Many factors need to be thoroughly evaluated when an athlete has chronic lower back pain. Degenerative arthritis, involvement of the lumbar spinal nerves and sacroiliac joint, and nonorthopedic pathology are a few of the many possible contributing factors.

Hip, Groin, and Pelvis

Chronic conditions at the hip frequently involve recurrent adductor or hip flexor strain. The involved muscle must be adequately strengthened and stretched. Chronic-phase strengthening exercises for this area are similar to those used in the subacute phase. The treatment emphasis should be on strengthening the hip flexor and on the adductor for chronic groin strain.

Knee

Acute and subacute knee conditions involving the ligamentous and cartilaginous structures are present in chronic cases as well. Another common condition is patellofemoral pain, for which (as pointed out in the previous chapter on ROM) stretching is important in managing. However, strengthening of the quadriceps is also required to protect the sore kneecap. Keep in mind that quadriceps strengthening must be designed specifically for each athlete experiencing patellofemoral pain.

For patellofemoral pain, pain-free quadriceps work is usually performed in the last 30° of extension (terminal knee extensions), but this is not always the case. Completely straightening the knee with a quadriceps contraction at 0° extension (with isometrics, straight-leg raise, or extension work) may increase kneecap pain. If this is the case, complete extension should be avoided.

Remember, any attempts to increase the strength of the quadriceps must be done without pain (for specific exercises, see Table 10.3).

In overuse injuries of the knee, the extensor mechanism can break down at the quadriceps tendon; at the junction of the quadriceps tendon and the superior pole of the patella (jumper's knee); at the inferior pole of the patella at its junction with the patellar tendon; at the patellar tendon itself (patellar tendinitis); or, in the growing athlete, at the tibial tubercle (Osgood-Schlatter's disease). Quadriceps strengthening exercises should be performed through the full ROM, if tolerated. Eccentric quadriceps work is particularly beneficial in patellar tendinitis and jumper's knee. These activities include slow, controlled lowering of the leg from complete knee extension. A progressive eccentric loading program using body weight as resistance can be helpful as well. Such a program should be instituted and monitored by trained specialists. Bounding (plyometrics) and jumping activities should be deemphasized until they can be performed pain free.

Calf, Ankle, and Foot

Ankle sprains can become chronic if not properly stretched and strengthened. Proper ankle sprain treatment was described in chapter 9 and in the section on subacute strengthening exercise in this chapter.

Other common chronic problems of the ankle and foot are Achilles tendinitis and plantar fasciitis. Stretching of the calf is essential for managing both of these problems, but strengthening can also play a helpful role. Toe raises that emphasize the eccentric component (lowering slowly from a tiptoe position to the starting position) are beneficial in managing Achilles tendinitis. Body weight resistance by the heel-drop method should be added only after consulting a sports medicine specialist.

Table 10.3
Strengthening Guidelines for Common Knee Conditions

Conditions	Activities to emphasize	Activities to avoid
Patellofemoral pain	Pain-free extension (usually terminal extension)	Heavy-loaded extension from 90° to 35°; squats; stair running
Anterior cruciate ligament tear	Midrange knee extension	Terminal extension from 40° to 0°
Partial	Knee flexion; external tibial rotation	
Complete	Full knee extension; knee flexion; external tibial rotation	. . .
Posterior cruciate ligament tear	Full knee extension	Heavy-loaded knee flexion
Meniscus tear		
Acute	Midrange knee extension	Terminal extension
Subacute	Full knee extension	Squats

Note. These are general strengthening guidelines for the proper management of common knee problems. This is not an all-inclusive listing, as all cases are unique and should be treated as such by a trained rehabilitation specialist.

Strengthening the intrinsic muscles of the foot may prove helpful in plantar fasciitis. Methods to strengthen the muscles that curl the toes (toe flexors) can be as simple as picking up a pencil or small objects (e.g., towel or marbles) from the floor with the toes (see Figure 10.8).

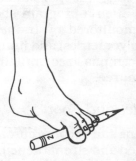

Figure 10.8. Pencil-curling exercise to strengthen toe flexor muscles.

CONCLUSION

Isolated, vigorous muscle strengthening is a key to effective sport rehabilitation. Incorrect, inappropriate, or inefficient strengthening exercises can be detrimental. I hope that this chapter adequately described both the difference between the two and how you can implement the former. Assuming that you have a good grasp of stretching and strengthening, it is appropriate to turn to another component addressed in effective sport rehabilitation: proprioception.

CHAPTER SUMMARY

1. Adequate muscle strength is a pre-requisite for sport participation. After injury, when strength is compromised, exercise to improve muscle strength is essential for efficient joint movement, muscle force generation, and dynamic joint stability.

2. Muscle contractions are either concentric (shortening), eccentric (lengthening), or isometric (muscle tension with no joint movement).

3. Concentric and eccentric muscle contractions that produce joint movement can be performed through the joint's ROM either isotonically or isokinetically.

4. Isotonic refers to constant resistance throughout the full ROM, whereas isokinetic refers to constant speed throughout full ROM.

5. Muscle tissue must be stressed gradually. A muscle will become stronger only if it is stressed to the point of exhaustion or momentary failure. Gradual overloading of the muscle is the most effective method of muscle strengthening.

6. In the sport rehabilitation strengthening program, more repetitions at low resistance should be performed early, progressing to fewer repetitions at higher resistance.

7. Biofeedback and functional electrical stimulation are two means of reeducating muscles in a sport rehabilitation program.

8. You can assist in this phase of rehabilitation by motivating your athletes during the strengthening program and watching for improper weight-lifting techniques.

Chapter 11
Exercises to Improve Proprioception

Proprioception, or joint sense, is the ability of a body part to signal the brain as to that joint's location in space. Joint sense is often overlooked in the traditional sport rehabilitation program even though a strong and flexible "smart" joint is the best protection against injury.

An athlete who has injured an ankle or a knee commonly complains that the affected joint "gives way." Factors such as muscle weakness and mechanical instability contribute to this subjective feeling. However, when injury rehabilitation addresses motion and strength deficiencies but not proprioception, the giving-way feeling often persists. Whether joint structures are intact or injury has compromised joint capsule, ligament, or other structures, proprioception is vital.

In this chapter, I describe proprioception and ways to address (in both prevention and rehabilitation) and assess proprioception. First, let's look at what is involved in normal proprioception.

THE PROPRIOCEPTION RESPONSE

Normal, controlled muscle function is a complex phenomenon. Receptors in the muscle and joint must provide information to higher brain centers to voluntarily and involuntarily fine tune movement. This feedback system must take into account not only coordination of a specific body part but also that body part's coordinated movement with the rest of the body.

For example, the athlete returning to the floor after rebounding a basketball must have adequate proprioception to allow the ankle to tell the brain whether the ankle is in good position to bear weight when it comes in contact with the floor and to line up the ankle with the knee, hip, and back to provide a stable, wide base so the player can safely absorb the impact of the body as the feet land on the court. And, if a joint, like the ankle, cannot tell the brain where that joint is in space quickly and accurately, the brain cannot tell the muscle how to adjust appropriately.

Mechanoreceptors provide joint sense and are located in the joint capsule and the ligaments that surround a joint. In cases of complete capsule and ligament disruption and subsequent mechanoreceptor damage, a joint may lose the ability to provide adequate information to the brain.

METHODS FOR ASSESSING ANKLE PROPRIOCEPTION

A common way to improve proprioception of the ankle is similar to the way in which proprioception is assessed, that is, using the modified single-leg balance. I describe this and other methods to assess ankle proprioception and then extend my description to means of improving ankle proprioception.

Single-Leg Balance

The ability to remain supported on one leg without losing balance is often used to measure proprioception. Many factors enter into this ability, namely, the status of higher brain centers (especially the cerebellum), muscle strength, and previous training. However, the single-leg stance is more frequently used to assess proprioception. Single-leg tests can be made more difficult by performing the test with the eyes shut or in the dark, thereby eliminating visual cues.

Force Plate Stand

Determining the length of time an athlete is able to stand on a flat surface without losing balance is a rather simplistic assessment approach. A more sophisticated method of proprioception measurement involves the use of a force plate. In this procedure, the athlete stands on the plate, which signals to a computer shifts in the athlete's center of gravity. The varying stresses on the weight-bearing foot indicate the sway of the body and can be quantified as they are sensed on the force plate and processed by a computer. Like the single-leg balance, the force plate stand is a static assessment.

Wobble Board Balance

More dynamic measurement tools that measure joint sense as well as muscle response are the wobble board, tilt board, or a modification of these. The wobble board is a circular surface that the athlete stands on (see Figure 11.1a). Underneath the sphere is a half sphere that makes balance difficult. The athlete attempts to maintain balance on the wobble board for as long as possible. The timed assessment can be made more dynamic and difficult by having the athlete balance on the board while trying to move the disk in a circular fashion clockwise and counterclockwise (see Figures 11.1b, c).

A wobble board can be easily constructed using a sheet of 3/4- or 1/2-inch plywood that is 2 feet in diameter. A half croquet ball is then anchored in the center of the board by a wood screw.

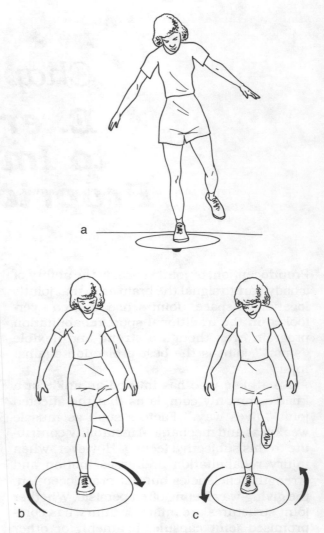

Figure 11.1. Wobble board activities to improve balance and proprioception: a, single-leg balance; b, clockwise motion; c, counterclockwise motion.

Tilt Board Technique

The tilt board procedure is also dynamic in that the athlete balances on the center of the board and alternately touches each side of the board on the floor. As performance improves, speed is increased so that the athlete is touching the floor with the board's sides as fast as possible. Like the wobble board, this technique requires not only static proprioception but also muscle power, strength, and quick reactions.

Instrumented tilt boards make quantification easier because the device automatically counts the number of times the edges touch the floor. A more sophisticated variation involves alternating flashing lights that are randomly activated by the machine as the athlete moves in the corresponding direction.

METHODS TO IMPROVE ANKLE PROPRIOCEPTION

Most research on proprioception as a factor to consider after joint injury has involved the ankle. In a flexible, strong ankle, much of the joint's stability is provided by the bones making up the joint. However, capsular, and especially ligamentous, support is vital as well, especially as the ankle is stressed in athletic activities.

Specific ways to improve proprioception are based on the same mechanics involved in assessing function.

Static Ankle Exercises

The athlete stands on a single leg with the arms out to the side (perpendicular to the trunk) and the elbows straight. At first, the eyes are kept open and the athlete is asked to maintain this position for 10 seconds before switching to the opposite leg.

As performance is mastered, the time that the athlete spends standing on the leg is decreased, making the switch from one leg to the other more rapid. A stable position is held for 3 to 5 seconds before switching.

Another approach, primarily for muscle endurance, is to have the athlete increase the amount of time spent standing on the affected side up to 5 to 10 minutes. After this stage is mastered, the athlete should perform the same technique with the arms down at the side, which serves to decrease the athlete's base of support. When this position is no longer difficult, the arms should be brought back up (again perpendicular to the trunk), but the athlete's eyes should be closed. The final step is to keep the eyes closed and bring the arms back down to the side.

Dynamic Ankle Exercises

When static standing is no longer difficult, resistance can be given to the athlete by a partner who gently attempts to push the athlete off balance. Resistance is given in all planes of motion and with increasing speed and intensity. Single-leg balance can also be stressed by having the athlete attempt to maintain balance while catching a tossed ball.

When these activities are easy, wobble board activities can be performed and progressed as in the single-leg drills. If simple balance on the wobble board is not difficult, the athlete can then try to touch the front, the back, and each side of the disk to the floor. Single touch can be progressed to trying to keep the edge about a half inch off the floor as the board is moved clockwise and counterclockwise.

Another modification that also stresses ankle strength can be performed by placing weights on the board. The BAPS board (biomechanical ankle platform system) is a useful tool for this purpose. Another helpful feature of the BAPS board is that you can change the size of the half sphere under the platform. As the training begins, a small half sphere is used before gradually progressing to a larger half sphere, making performance more difficult (see Figure 11.2).

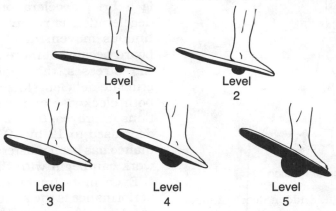

Level 1   Level 2   Level 3   Level 4   Level 5

Figure 11.2.   BAPS board.

METHODS TO IMPROVE KNEE PROPRIOCEPTION

Anterior cruciate ligament injury is one of the most frequently occurring and studied injuries in sport. Forces that disrupt this ligament in sports occur in thousandths of a second, but muscles cannot respond to protect the joint until after about half a second. Furthermore, as athletes get bigger and quicker, the forces exerted on this knee ligament increase.

However, as the incidence of this injury continues to rise, methods to maximize rehabilitation efforts have become more sophisticated and thorough. And, although research shows that strong quadriceps and supranormal hamstring strength are important, proprioception is also essential. For non-anterior-cruciate knee injuries, the progression of activities found in the previous section on the ankle is sufficient. However, to understand the goals of a proprioception program specific for the anterior cruciate-deficient athlete, you must first understand the functional instability that the program attempts to minimize.

Functional Instability of the Knee

Noncontact injury resulting in a torn anterior cruciate ligament is often caused by a sudden deceleration on the planted leg, usually with a twist. This maneuver also results in the knee giving way after the cruciate is torn. This giving-way phenomenon is referred to as a *pivot shift* (see Figure 11.3).

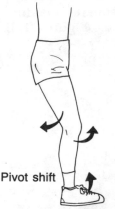

Pivot shift

Leg in internal rotation

Figure 11.3. Pivot shift. Sudden deceleration, especially with a simultaneous twisting motion, can result in anterior cruciate ligament rupture.

What happens in the cruciate-deficient knee is this. As the athlete quickly stops without the support of the cruciate, the tibia slides forward on the femur. Specifically, the outer (lateral) top portion of the tibia (tibial plateau) slides forward as the knee is close to extension. As the athlete's body continues forward over the fixed foot, the knee flexes, at which time the subluxated tibial plateau moves back to its normal position. The return of the tibia to this more normal position produces the giving-way sensation experienced by the anterior cruciate-deficient athlete.

Increasing Knee Stability

The goal of the proprioception program for the anterior cruciate-deficient knee is to allow the athlete to subconsciously or consciously control pivot shift. Pivot shift control requires hamstring activation that minimizes the forward motion of the tibia from underneath the femur.

Vital to pivot shift stability in the cruciate-deficient knee is control of the hamstrings. In short, if the knee rehabilitation program is to be successful, the athlete must be able to control the pivot shift by hamstring activation. This skill is sometimes automatic, but at other times is very difficult for the athlete to master. A trained medical specialist should oversee the progression of proprioception activities designed for the anterior cruciate-injured athlete.

Stationary single-leg activities are good drills to start with. When ready for dynamic activities, the athlete can use a 14-by-14 inch wobble board with half a croquet ball anchored to the bottom. The square disk is preferred because as each corner touches the floor there is a brief deceleration of the board. This deceleration is recommended over the continuous movement allowed by the circular board because it more effectively reproduces the stresses that endanger the anterior cruciate-deficient knee. As performance in both clockwise and counterclockwise directions improves, the size of the square can be decreased to 12 by 12 inches. When performance has been mastered with the eyes open, work can begin with the eyes closed.

Even more important than wobble-board performance is the athlete's ability to perform sport-specific maneuvers. This is especially true for the cruciate-deficient athlete. Advanced function testing and instructions are addressed in chapter 13.

METHODS TO IMPROVE SHOULDER PROPRIOCEPTION

Proprioceptive deficits are not always apparent after most arm injuries. The exception to this is shoulder dislocation. And, for athletes who throw or whose sport entails weight bearing on the upper extremities (e.g., gymnastics and wrestling), shoulder dislocation can be a real dilemma.

The earlier the age at which an athlete encounters the first dislocation, the greater the chances for subsequent dislocation. As the shoulder tends to dislocate, each reinjury causes further damage. It is important for the athlete to strengthen the muscles that assist in keeping the humeral head in an optimal, centralized position in the glenoid cavity. But it is similarly important to establish an intact feedback loop that tells the muscles how stable the shoulder is so the muscles can move the shoulder appropriately (proprioception).

Weight bearing facilitates joint proprioception. That's why efforts to improve knee and ankle stability employ exercises and activities that are performed in standing positions. Eventually, these activities progress to weight bearing (standing) on the involved side only.

The shoulder should be similarly stressed. Initial activities should require weight bearing on the arm, but these should not excessively stress the involved part of the capsule. Most frequently, the athlete who suffers frequent shoulder dislocations has a lax anterior capsule. This laxity may also affect other areas of the shoulder, namely the inferior and posterior capsules. Positions that athletes should avoid when loading or bearing weight on these three shoulder structures are shown in Table 11.1.

When bearing weight on both arms is no longer difficult, the athlete can begin assuming positions that allow weight bearing on the involved side only. Balance on the involved upper extremity can be facilitated by having the athlete use the appropriate arm to reach, catch, or strike an object while bearing weight solely on the involved arm.

Usually, there is no generalized instability of the shoulder after injury. Rather, it is more common for the shoulder to be positionally or functionally unstable; that is, the shoulder

Table 11.1
Precautions in Upper Extremity Loading and Weight Bearing

Shoulder site	Activities to avoid
Anterior	Flexed-elbow weight bearing (e.g., chest-to-ground starting push-up position); extremes of horizontal abduction (e.g., bar-to-chest bench pressing or extremes of fly or butterfly pectoral strengthening)
Posterior	Straight-elbow weight bearing (e.g., locked-elbow finish position with push-ups or bench press); extremes of horizontal adduction (e.g., elbow across chest assisted by opposite hand pulling arm closer to chest)
Inferior	Straight-elbow overhead weight bearing (e.g., finish position of overhead military press or head-standing wall push-ups)

"goes out" or "feels loose" only in a specific position, which is readily apparent only with a specific function.

The most common example is a baseball pitcher who complains of an arm losing power at the end of the cocking phase, just before the arm accelerates to deliver the ball. This so-called dead-arm syndrome is usually caused by anterior instability of the shoulder. A trained specialist should examine the shoulder to find the specific point of instability or positional weakness. Once the position is isolated, proprioceptive exercises that allow the athlete to use the rotator cuff muscles to maintain a stable location within the glenoid cavity should be used. After the athlete can find this position, strengthening exercises and then sport-specific activities should be progressed in this position.

CONCLUSION

Proprioception is a vital step toward regaining adequate function. And, in reality, strength and proprioception go hand in hand. A joint will be able to protect itself from abnormal forces only if it is both strong and smart. The total treatment program must also address flexibility. General guidelines for stretches that are appropriate for many common conditions are given in Appendix B.

CHAPTER SUMMARY

1. An intact feedback loop that allows a given joint to tell the brain where the joint is located in space (proprioception) is vital if that joint is to move as signaled by the brain.
2. Mechanoreceptors are located in joint capsule tissue and in ligaments that provide stability to a given joint. When capsular or ligamentous restraints are disrupted by athletic injury, proprioception can become impaired.
3. Bearing weight on the involved joint is essential for an athlete to reestablish proprioceptive feedback.
4. When injury results in joint instability, proprioceptive work is essential to teach the athlete normal and abnormal joint positions.

Chapter 12

Protective Devices, Padding, and Supports

Protective equipment has evolved immensely over the course of the last few years. Modern equipment not only protects better but also fits the athlete more closely and comfortably than did equipment used in years past.

Protective equipment is a major factor in decreasing injury. If you doubt this, look at the dramatic decrease in eye injuries sustained by ice hockey players after rules of the sport were changed to require helmets and face masks. The purpose of this section, however, is not to discuss the required and customary protective padding for a given sport. I assume that your athletes already wear all the standard equipment for your specific sport.

So, instead, this chapter focuses on the braces, wraps, splints, pads, and other equipment specifically used after injury. These protective devices range from simple, cheap common-sense interventions to sophisticated, expensive, complex fittings.

Protective splinting, bracing, and padding can indeed be vital adjuncts to the sport rehabilitation process; and judicious use of such protective devices may give the rehabilitated athlete an edge. But such measures alone are not an answer. Also, they are not a remedy for the nonrehabilitated athlete.

FUNCTIONS OF PROTECTIVE EQUIPMENT

Devices used in addition to the usual protective equipment such as braces, wraps, and pads serve several functions. Protection is afforded the involved body part as these pieces of equipment

- deflect forces away from the injury,
- absorb forces directed at the injury, and
- limit movement.

Deflect Forces

Forces can be deflected or transferred to another structure or body part by soft or hard protective pads. For example, a runner with a bunion on the big toe can deflect the forces away from the area with a soft "donut" pad that decreases friction over the involved soft tissue.

Absorb Forces

Energy can also be effectively absorbed by placing a pad over an injured area. An example of this is a football player with a bruise to the upper arm. If the area is not adequately covered by the shoulder pads, a special pad can be fabricated and placed over the area so that contact is harmlessly absorbed.

Limit Movement

Excessive motion can be controlled by splinting, bracing, or taping. Examples of protective equipment providing this function include traditional ankle taping and other modes of taping and wrapping that protect an area by limiting motion.

TYPES OF PROTECTIVE EQUIPMENT

The following descriptions of the types, application, and composition of protective equipment should help you understand how your athletes may benefit by using them.

Braces

A brace is an external device usually applied at a joint to limit ROM. Certain nonthreatening motions are allowed by bracing, but movements stressing injured structures are minimized or prevented.

Materials

Braces geared to withstand high-impact forces and limit motion significantly in a given plane have a nonyielding component. Generally speaking, if ROM is to be limited, the brace should be made of more rigid material and be custom made for proper fit. Common structures used in sport braces are steel, aluminum or aluminum alloy, graphite, and high-density plastics. Limitations in motion are created by the high tensile strength of the materials used in the brace or built-in, adjustable ROM stops (dials, springs, straps, etc.). Other, less rigid braces are made of lighter plastics, canvas, or nylon straps. These braces provide limited support and need not be specifically sized and fitted.

Of special concern regarding bracing is a particular brace's legality in a given sport. Certain sport-governing bodies allow bracing, whereas others do not. Some braces with a protective covering worn over the brace are allowed, but in other cases the brace is not allowed even with protective covering. It is wise to check with sport officials before a brace is purchased and utilized by the athlete to see whether the brace can be worn legally.

Cost

Some low-cost braces function well, but rigid, customized braces can be quite costly. For ex-

ample, braces commonly used after knee injury can range from $300 to $500. Therefore, the cost-benefit issue should be thoroughly discussed with the athlete before fitting the athlete with a brace.

Padding

Additional padding over an injured area is applied to absorb and transmit force from the involved area. This additional padding serves as an adjunct to any existing, normal padding worn by the athlete in a particular sport. Padding can be soft and yielding, or it can be firm, rigid, and unyielding. Adjunctive padding can be used with normal padding for a sport (e.g., soft padding worn underneath football shoulder pads) or can be used separately from routine protective equipment (e.g., elbow pads).

Materials

There is a wide variety of materials available for soft and hard protective padding. Common materials used for soft padding are foam rubber, self-adhesive foam rubber, orthopedic felt, Viscolas, PPT, Ensolite, and Plastizote. These materials are of different densities and thicknesses and absorb shock to varying degrees. Hard protective padding is usually made of a high density plastic, polypropylene, or a similar material.

Pads can effectively cover the entire involved area by maintaining contact with the surface to be protected (e.g., soft foam rubber padding placed in a shoe for a painful heel bruise). Or, bubble pads can be used to guard the affected area by maintaining contact around the periphery and bubbling up over the painful area, thus eliminating direct pressure on the injury site.

Securing a pad can be difficult at times. One way to make the pad conform to the involved body part is to use a heat-sensitive material. Plastizote is a very practical option for soft padding, whereas Orthoplast is a desirable material for rigid padding. Plastizote can be heated in an oven to a temperature that renders it very pliable, so that it can be molded into the desired shape or contour. As the Plastizote cools, the material maintains the new shape. Similarly, Orthoplast produces the same effect in a rigid form after it is heated in hot water. Once a pad is fabricated, it can be held in place by a wrap, a neoprene sleeve, or an elastic stockinette or may be attached to another piece of equipment (e.g., secured to shoulder pads).

Splints

A splint is an external support designed to immobilize an injured area. The splint protects and immobilizes like a cast, but it can be removed more easily. Splints are commonly used to limit motion of an acutely injured body part and then are discarded as the injury heals and strength and ROM improve.

However, immobilization may need to be continued to allow sufficient healing of an injury, even after pain has gone and strength and ROM are at functional levels. This may create a dilemma for the coach, athlete, and sports medicine specialist. Should the athlete be allowed to play if he or she is completely healed and has no pain, sufficient strength, and full ROM? If the athlete can compete safely, the answer is yes. If the rules permit splints and casts and if adequate protection is afforded the involved body part, participation can be allowed. Adequate protection means that the joint or body part is appropriately immobilized without jeopardizing another body part or risking injury to another participant.

Materials

Splinting, when allowed, should be done with a nonyielding material such as plaster, fiberglass, or heat-moldable plastics (e.g., Orthoplast or Orofit). Certain sports and governing bodies allow these materials as long as they are padded. Other sports and organizations, on the other hand, forbid the use of such materials for competition.

You should know the rules specific to your sport regarding splinting, so periodically check with the national governing body or state organization that sets up and enforces the rules to assure compliance.

Taping

Perhaps every coach at every level has at one time wrestled with a roll of tape. But taping is not the mysterious secret some make it out to be. Taping is like any other skill in that the more the skill is performed, the more profi-

cient one becomes in performing the skill. Tape is used in athletic injuries to secure a dressing, to assist in holding a pad in place, or most often to provide additional support to an injured or weak area.

Questions about taping revolve around the amount of support that tape offers and whether taping renders a joint weak and thus makes the joint (or others close to it) more susceptible to injury. This book examines these issues only in relation to specific body parts. Many fine textbooks are available that you and other coaches can consult for more information on taping and that explain proper skin preparation, step-by-step taping techniques, and so on. But here are a few basic principles for you to keep in mind:

- Make sure to properly position the body part to be taped.
- Never tape a body part as a quick fix, and always thoroughly evaluate an injury before taping.
- Remember that taping is an adjunct to the treatment program and not a substitute for adequate motion, strength, and proprioception.
- Leave taping to a competent individual with appropriate skill and experience. The best intentions in applying a tape job can be negated if the tape is applied incorrectly and results in reinjury, tape cuts that subsequently become infected, or major skin irritation.

Materials

Use the appropriate kind of tape for the job. When more support is required, complement the use of standard adhesive-backed cloth tape with high-tensile tape (Elasticon or moleskin). When less support is needed or when swelling is present, an elastic adhesive tape (Conform or J Flex) may be appropriate.

Wraps

A wrap is used when circumferential compression around an area is needed to disperse force from an injured area. A wrap is applied around an involved joint or muscle belly to provide warmth, to secure a pad, or to minimally restrict extremes of joint movement.

Materials

Common wraps are elastic bandages, neoprene sleeves, and elastic stockinettes. The elastic component allows for muscle excursion and joint movement without restricting or compromising function to a large degree. When elastic bandages are used around a body part, tension should be sufficient to provide support but not restrict blood flow. If the athlete's skin becomes discolored below the wrap or if the athlete complains of a cool or numb feeling below the wrap, the wrap is too tight. Also, when wrapping the body part circumferentially, apply the wrap in a diagonal rather than a circular manner.

PROTECTIVE EQUIPMENT FOR SPECIFIC BODY PARTS

With a general knowledge of the various types of protective devices, let's examine how these devices protect specific body parts after common sport injuries.

Neck

Adequate stabilization of the head and neck after acute injury is paramount. Because the athlete must be able to move the neck freely for visual awareness, bracing of the neck is not a realistic option. Semirigid support that significantly prohibits neck ROM is also not practical.

Neck Collars

Still, some neck-protecting alternatives remain. For example, neck rolls are often used in contact sports, particularly in football. A neck collar or neck roll is frequently worn by athletes who have sustained repeated stingers or burners. Commercially available neck rolls that attach to the shoulder pads directly below the helmet are frequently worn by football players to restrict undesired excessive motion. The thick, triangular-shaped wedge pad restricts extension but does not significantly affect rotation or lateral flexion of the cervical spine. A neck roll that leaves only the front of the neck open is also routinely used to limit excessive lateral flexion.

Often, commercially available collars do not sufficiently cradle the neck and thus allow excessive motion. In such cases, a self-made collar may be more effective. For example, you might roll up an appropriately sized piece of Ensolite and place it in a 2- or 3-inch-diameter stockinette. This roll conforms to the athlete's neck much better. Once the roll is in proper position, the excess length of stockinette is looped through the shoulder pads (one end under and the other end on top of the shoulder pad) and tied in front.

Shoulder and Shoulder Girdle

The shoulder, the most mobile joint in the body, is frequently injured in sports. Contact sports report many shoulder injuries, but numerous injuries are reported in noncontact sports as well.

Shoulder Padding

In contact sports, some type of shoulder padding is a standard part of the uniform with a few exceptions (e.g., rugby). Protective padding is also often used to disperse force from injured shoulders. And, injuries to the clavicle, sternoclavicular, and acromioclavicular joints may require additional padding. For less tender conditions, a commercially available half-inch-foam, lace-up pad can be worn under the regular shoulder pads. When this does not adequately protect the area, custom-made Orthoplast bubble pads are very useful. Self-adhesive foam can then be applied to the part of the pad that is in contact with the athlete to absorb shock. Contusions can also be protected by custom-made or commercially available pads.

Shoulder Taping

When additional support or restricted motion is the primary goal, taping techniques may be employed. Sprains of the sternoclavicular and acromioclavicular joints, as well as glenohumeral subluxation and dislocation, are common conditions that may require additional support.

When taping for sternoclavicular and acromioclavicular sprains, adequate adherence of the tape to the skin may be a problem.

The injured joint must be taped in the proper, stable position. Such taping procedures may require more resilient tape than the standard white, adhesive-backed cloth tape.

Shoulder Bracing

Tape, however, is not effective in maintaining stability of the glenohumeral joint in cases of recurrent shoulder subluxation or dislocation. Control of glenohumeral motion requires that arm movement be restricted to prevent potentially compromising positions of the shoulder. Standard tape would likely rip or present difficulties in "connecting" the arm with the trunk to provide sufficient protection. Therefore, an elastic bandage with an elasticized tape should be properly wrapped around the shoulder in an attempt to control dislocation.

An even more effective means of protecting shoulder dislocations is the commercially available canvas and rope braces that prevent the shoulder from moving into vulnerable positions. Also available is a much more sophisticated model brace that has a high-density plastic shell and is form fit to the athlete's trunk and upper arm. Such braces allow shoulder motion in a protected range only. These braces are relatively expensive but may be a worthwhile consideration in certain cases.

Elbow, Wrist, and Hand

Because nearly every sport requires athletes to grasp, catch, pull, strike, throw, and push with their upper extremities, injury to the elbow, wrist, and hands is common. But bracing, padding, wrapping, and splinting of upper extremities must provide adequate support without restricting function. This is especially tricky when dealing with the fingers and hands, as fine-tuned hand movement is necessary to perform the precise and coordinated upper extremity motions involved in throwing, racket, and swinging sports.

Elbow Bracing

Tennis elbow may require bracing. Counterforce bracing will help decrease the discomfort of this condition, which is often experienced by racket-sport players. An example of counterforce bracing is the neoprene sleeve. Worn around the origin of the wrist flexors and extensors and supported by a strap, the neoprene sleeve is a very effective device for this elbow condition.

Elbow, Wrist, and Hand Taping

Commercially available neoprene sleeves, worn around the upper and lower arm and connected by a nylon webbing strap, can be adjusted to help check elbow hyperextension. After elbow sprain or rehabilitated dislocation, tape is used to help prevent undesired motion. Standard white adhesive-backed cloth tape should be reinforced by a heavy-duty tape.

Wrist and finger sprains and strains are also frequently taped. However, the trick here is to provide adequate protection while still allowing the athlete as much hand function as possible.

Elbow, Wrist, and Hand Splinting

Although fractures are usually thought of as absolute contraindications to sport participation, some athletes with wrist or forearm fractures, as well as severe hand sprains or fractures, can compete if the injury is casted or splinted. And, although casting is something you, as a coach, will not do, you should be aware of all options when situations require casting or splinting.

In some sports, casts and splints are allowed if they are covered adequately by soft padding. In cases in which rigid support is illegal, silicone "casts" are used. These form-fit casts provide the immobilization offered by a regular cast or splint, but, because they are soft and yielding, they are legal in certain sports in which rigid support is not permitted. Heat-molded soft padding (Plastizote) can be used for protection when the immobilization offered by plaster or fiberglass is not needed. Splinting material that can be molded to the shape of the body part (Orthoplast) also affords suitable protection. Thinner strips of a similar moldable material (Orofit) work exceptionally well with finger and hand splinting.

Hand Padding

Soft-padding techniques are also frequently used in managing bruises of the hand. Thin, high-density padding (PPT) is especially good for this purpose. Soft pads can be taped on the hand or incorporated inside a glove.

Lower Back

Lumbar strains, sprains, and contusions are often incurred by the athlete. Warmth is often soothing for lower back strain or sprain. Heat allows muscles to stretch easier and prevents the back from tightening up in cold outdoor temperatures.

Back Supports

Neoprene back supports are one way to keep the lower back warm. Such lower back supports are wrapped around the trunk and held in place by Velcro straps. More sophisticated supports have additional strapping configurations that provide even greater security. Some of these supports also contain a broad sheet of Orthoplast, which can be molded to the shape of the back and inserted inside the sleeve. Such form-fit back supports provide minimal restriction of motion yet offer more resistance to extension than the simple neoprene sleeve.

Back Bracing

In cases of stress fracture of the lower back or other conditions in which lumbar hyperextension must be limited, athletes can compete if they use a functional form of lumbar immobilization. A high-density, heat-molded, form-fitted brace can be used successfully and safely. This type of brace must be made by a trained brace maker (orthotist) and is usually quite expensive.

Hip, Groin, and Pelvis

Athletes in contact sports rarely need additional support and padding of the hip area because such equipment is usually included in their uniforms. However, a significant fall or blow can cause injury even to a padded area. And hip injury is always possible in activities in which padding is not used.

Hip Padding

One extremely painful injury to the hip is the hip pointer, a bruise to the iliac crest of the pelvis (see Figure 12.1). Because there is usually little soft-tissue protection over this area, the bone is susceptible to direct trauma.

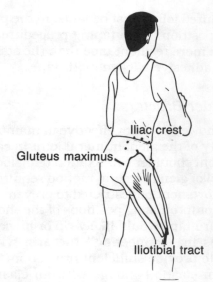

Figure 12.1.   Hip pointer.

When additional padding is required, a soft-backed bubble pad of Orthoplast usually works well. The pad can be held in place by an elastic wrap or can be incorporated into an existing article of the athlete's uniform. Elastic "sliding shorts" or bicycling shorts are also convenient ways to apply a pad to this area.

A problem similar to the hip pointer is experienced at the greater torchanter of the femur. In such cases, comparable padding measures should be used.

Hip and Groin Wrapping

Elastic wraps and tape are sometimes used after groin strain to help provide warmth and extra support for the involved muscle or to help restrict motion. When warmth or support is desired, an elastic wrap or neoprene groin sleeve is appropriate. If restriction of motion is necessary, the hip must be wrapped with the injured muscle in a shortened position. For a hip flexor strain, the hip should be slightly flexed and the elastic wrap or tape pulled toward hip flexion (see Figure 12.2).

When the adductors are involved, the hip should be held in a position slightly toward the opposite leg as the tape or wrap is applied, and the wrap should be pulled toward the opposite leg (see Figure 12.3).

Thigh

Serious quadriceps damage can result from inadvertent contact or prior slight muscle strain.

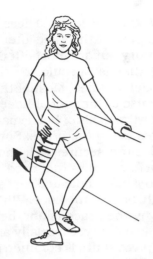

Figure 12.2. Elastic wrap for hip flexor strain.

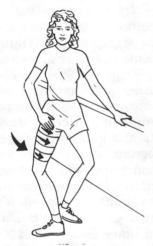

Figure 12.3. Elastic wrap for hip adductor strain.

If damaged, quadriceps muscle mass is more easily injured by excessive exertion or blunt trauma than is normally resilient, properly functioning muscle tissue.

Thigh Padding

Thigh padding is standard equipment in some sports in which contact is likely, and protective padding is an absolute must for an athlete who has suffered a severe quadriceps strain or contusion. But blunt trauma to the thigh will still cause or exacerbate injury if the padding provides inadequate coverage or support. Additional and properly applied padding, therefore, is necessary to help prevent further damage by blunt trauma.

In football, commercially available thigh pads are used to cover a larger area and provide more protection than standard thigh pads. In sports in which thigh padding is not normally used, a football thigh pad or custom-fit Orthoplast bubble pad can be used. The protective pad must be held securely in place yet still allow for quadriceps muscle function. Elastic wraps often slide down the leg or allow the pad to slip, so a neoprene thigh sleeve may be a better alternative for securing such protective pads.

Thigh Wrapping

Other soft-tissue thigh injuries also respond positively to the additional support provided by a neoprene sleeve. Proximal (upper) hamstring strains can be supported effectively by a neoprene groin sleeve wrapped high around the groin area. Distal (lower) hamstring strains are aided by an open-patella knee sleeve, whereas mid-muscle-belly strains of the hamstrings can benefit from the support offered by a neoprene thigh sleeve.

Knee

In this section, I first examine ways to protect the patella and extensor mechanism (quadriceps and patellar tendon) and then discuss protective padding and bracing for ligament and cartilage problems.

Patella Wrapping

Warmth, rather than compression, is often desired in various overuse injuries around the knee. Thus, open-patella knee sleeves have been quite useful in protecting conditions such as quadriceps tendinitis, patellar tendinitis, and synovitis.

Patella Padding

Bruised areas around the kneecap, as well as the adolescent suffering from Osgood-Schlatter's disease, need some form of knee protection. Commercially available heavy-duty knee pads (similar to volleyball pads) may be adequate. But in cases in which extra protection is needed, a small Orthoplast bubble pad placed over the involved area and held in place by an open-patella neoprene sleeve works well.

Another soft-tissue problem that often requires rigid protection is *prepatellar bursitis*. Although reported in other sports, prepatellar bursitis is a condition most common to wrestlers. Consistent friction to the anterior (front) of the knee causes the bursa between the skin and the patella to become inflamed. When the athlete is able to compete, protection against further excessive friction should be provided. This is difficult to do without restricting knee ROM. An Orthoplast bubble pad is the best form of protection for this problem but is difficult to fabricate.

Patella Bracing

Bracing to provide restraint to excessive patellar movement can be helpful in managing patellar subluxation, patellar dislocation, and patellofemoral pain syndrome. Many types of these braces are available, most of which include an elastic or neoprene sleeve with a buttress that restricts movement of the patella.

Whether to use a patella brace depends on the clinician and the preference of the athlete. Important considerations are the location, consistency, and support offered by the patellar buttress and the weight, comfort, and fit of the sleeve.

Patella Taping

Taping to dynamically assist in maintaining patellar position may effectively decrease patellofemoral pain. However, this taping procedure requires advanced training and should be left to a sports medicine specialist.

Knee Braces

Bracing or taping the knee after cartilage or ligament injury or using a brace to "prevent" knee injury are presently some of the most debated topics in sports medicine.

Knee braces that protect the knee after surgery are beyond the scope of this book. So this discussion focuses on knee bracing that supports or precludes injury to knee ligaments and cartilage.

Knee braces are classified into three categories:

- Functional
- Prophylactic
- Rehabilitation (worn after surgery and not discussed here)

Functional knee braces.   These braces are designed to protect the knee after all types of ligament injury but are most often thought of as bracing that is specific for the anterior cruciate-deficient knee. Most of the data supporting the use of functional knee braces are subjective testimonials of brace manufacturers or of athletes using the brace. Some athletes simply feel more secure with the knee in a brace. But a few studies that used more objective measures have indicated that such braces may actually benefit the knee. Which athletes are helped by the brace is another question.

Rotatory instability, especially anterolateral instability (pivot shift), is common after injury to the anterior cruciate ligament. The pivot shift phenomenon is the functional instability that negatively affects performance in the anterior cruciate-deficient athlete. Functional knee braces try to control the rotatory instability by intricate cam systems, bars on the brace, plastic or graphite shells butting against the tibia, elastic straps, or any combination of these.

Even with adequate hamstring strength, appropriate quadriceps-to-body ratios, appropriate hamstring-to-quadriceps ratios, sufficient proprioception, and a sound functional progression program, some athletes will still pivot shift or demonstrate functional instability during sport activity. In my opinion, these are the athletes who should be braced. If the athlete is not willing to give up a particular sport and can afford a brace that costs $300 to $600, then bracing may be an option before surgery.

Prophylactic knee braces.   Another type of knee brace commonly used in sport is the lateral, or prophylactic, knee brace. Designed primarily to prevent injury resulting from a blow to the outside (lateral aspect) of the knee, this brace has been a source of controversy for some time (see Figure 12.4).

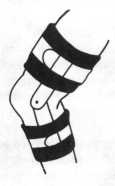

Figure 12.4.   Prophylactic lateral knee brace.

The Unhappy Triad of O'Donoghue

In contact sports, "The Unhappy Triad of O'Donoghue" used to be the most frequently reported mechanism of injury to the anterior cruciate ligament. This sequence of events was named after a pioneer sports orthopedist, Dr. Don O'Donoghue, who initially described the injury.

An illegal clip block on a football player produced excessive force at the lateral knee, causing a valgus stress and placing stress on the medial collateral ligament. The force was too great and thus tore the medial collateral ligament (first injury of the triad sequence). Additional force then tore the medial meniscus (second injury of the triad). Finally, the anterior cruciate ligament was torn because of the stress from previous events in O'Donoghue's triad (see Figure 12.5).

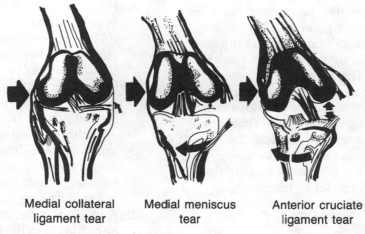

Medial collateral
ligament tear

Medial meniscus
tear

Anterior cruciate
ligament tear

Figure 12.5.   The Unhappy Triad of O'Donoghue.

It was postulated that a lateral knee brace would absorb the force of a blow and prevent this mechanism of injury from occurring. Suddenly, it seemed that everyone was manufacturing lateral knee braces. A series of studies were performed to determine the effectiveness of the braces. Initial results indicated that the brace preloaded (stretched) the medial collateral ligament and thus increased the risk of injury. Further research showed that bearing weight negated the preloading effect demonstrated in the laboratory. More recent studies involving large numbers of football players show conflicting data.

Among the other factors to consider in deciding whether to use lateral knee braces to prevent injury are the cost of the braces (approximately $100 to $150 a pair), proper fit, and placement of the brace.

Calf, Ankle, and Foot

Injuries to the ankle and foot, even if they are not serious, can severely hamper the function of an athlete. Even the tiniest blister or bunion on a toe can make walking difficult and running virtually impossible. Taping and padding the injured ankle and foot can be an effective part of an injury management program.

Calf, Ankle, and Foot Padding

Contusions of the calf, ankle, and foot can be effectively padded in a variety of ways. Orthoplast bubble pads are quite useful in protecting against further trauma to calf bruises.

Deep calf bruises and severe, blunt trauma to the shin can be very serious. And, even after motion and strength have returned, extra protection is vital. Soft padding is sometimes enough, but rigid protection is frequently required. The pads can be held in place by elastic wraps, elastic stockinettes, or neoprene calf sleeves.

Padding the foot can be especially difficult because there must be sufficient room for the athlete to get a shoe on over the pad. High-density, thin, soft padding (PPT or Viscolas) may work.

Ankle Bracing and Taping

When motion of the foot or ankle must be restricted, many options are available. Adhesive-backed athletic tape has been used for the ankle for many years. A good tape job initially offers adequate immobilization of the injured ankle, but it loosens significantly as the athlete puts stress on the tape.

Therefore, a lace-up ankle support may be preferred over tape. This brace provides more support for a longer period of time than does tape. After injury it is wise to use both the lace-up brace and tape. Be cautious, however, in choosing an ankle brace because quality fluctuates greatly from model to model.

Foot Taping

Various tape jobs have been successful in supplying extra support for foot and toe conditions. The use of tape to limit excessive pronation of the foot has been effective in helping to manage complaints of shin splints. However, when additional, long-term support is needed to control excessive, abnormal foot movement or to more normally distribute forces on the foot, an orthotic may be helpful.

In this case, an *orthotic* is any object placed inside the shoe to help support or protect the foot. Orthotics range from the inexpensive,

soft insert to the sophisticated, expensive ones. Heel lifts can aid in helping to manage early Achilles tendinitis, Sever's disease, and plantar fasciitis. Heel lifts or heel cups also help to decrease pain from heel bruises or heel pad inflammation. Although orthotics are not the panacea that some people make them out to be, they may help manage foot disorders that result in dysfunction at the knee, hip, and all the way up to the lower back.

CHAPTER SUMMARY

1. Protective equipment, padding, and bracing serve important adjunctive roles by preventing sport injury to tissue that is healthy and by supporting tissue that has been previously injured.
2. Protective equipment, padding, and bracing protect involved body parts by deflecting or transmitting forces, absorbing or dispersing energy, and limiting undesirable excessive motion, respectively. Padding can be rigid or soft and either incorporated into existing padding or used alone.
3. A brace is most often used in sport rehabilitation to limit excessive motion at a joint. More sophisticated rigid bracing must be checked for compliance with the rules and regulations of the sport.
4. Splints used in sport rehabilitation are designed to provide significant immobilization of an injured body part. Although the splinting is usually applied during the acute injury phase when the athlete is not participating, some splints can be safely used during athletic competition.

Chapter 13

Functional Progression: Returning to Activity

So now your athlete's injury is rehabilitated. Active ROM is full, equal with the opposite side, or within normal limits for a given body part. Muscle strength is normal. Muscle endurance is acceptable. Pain is absent. Swelling is also gone. The involved area has been braced, padded, or taped appropriately. The athlete is ready to return to competition and full participation, right? Wrong!

The athlete must first reestablish sport-specific function. And a game situation is no place to determine whether the athlete's function after injury is up to competitive standards. That is why functional progression is such an important part of sport rehabilitation.

Functional progression is a sport-specific program in which movement patterns required in a given sport are progressed according to the difficulty of the skill and the athlete's tolerance of the activities. This part of the rehabilitation process is often neglected, only to have the athlete reinjured.

No person is better able to evaluate one of your athlete's performance of sport-specific activities than you, the coach. You also are capable of monitoring your athlete's improvement during the functional progression program. Your insight into the specifics of your sport, combined with a personal relationship with your athletes, gives you the potential to be a tremendous asset in this stage of sport rehabilitation. But, before you can help, you must fully understand the basics of functional progression and the benefits of a functional progression program.

BASIC PRINCIPLES OF FUNCTIONAL PROGRESSION

Function progression is a series of sport-specific, basic movement patterns that are gradually progressed according to the difficulty of the skill and the athlete's tolerance. These movement patterns are broken down and progressed from simple to complex until the athlete has regained preinjury function.

Laws of Healing

Injured tissue heals according to the stresses placed on the involved structures. For example, a cut over the knuckle of a finger heals over, and a scab is produced. As the finger bends, stresses at the knuckle cause the scab to open up. Eventually, the cut heals completely, and new, pliable skin allows free motion at the site. The skin healed according to the stresses that were placed on it during the healing phase.

The same thing happens when bones, ligaments, and tendons heal. Consistent with Wolff's law, bone heals according to the stresses placed on it. After bone is injured, new bone growth is stimulated according to the manner in which it is stressed. Furthermore, Davis's law states that healing soft tissue responds to stresses placed on it by becoming more resistant to forces along the direction of the applied stress.

The principles behind Wolff's and Davis's laws are also important concepts of functional progression. If an athlete is not ready to accept the physical demands of the sport in which his or her injury occurred, injury will likely recur. Functional progression avoids this outcome by first breaking down required sport-specific movement patterns and then progressively reinitiating them according to the athlete's tolerance and performance of the skills.

For example, a basketball player recuperating from a sprained ankle can regain motion and strength by performing ROM and strengthening exercises during the rehabilitation process. These exercises are designed to stress the healing ligaments of the ankle as it progresses through active and then resisted full ROM. According to Davis's law, the stress placed on the healing ligaments during AROM causes the ligaments to become stronger.

Basketball, however, demands more of the ankle than motion in a single axis and against controlled resistance. During the course of a basketball game, an athlete must be able to withstand superimposed body weight, sprinting, stopping, cutting, jumping, hopping, and other movements. Again, according to Davis's law, these activities should be performed before actually competing to stress the healing ligaments and strengthen them. A well-planned functional progression for this basketball player would ensure that healing ankle structures are stressed gradually to ready them for the demands of basketball. Without functional progression, the healing tissues will not be stressed sufficiently to maximize sport readiness.

Principle of Preparedness

At the heart of functional progression is the "SAID" principle (Specific Adaptations to Imposed Demands). This means that the treatment principles of functional progression must be specific not only to the sport but also to the demands placed on an athlete performing a given function in that sport.

Functional progression must be tailored to each athlete. So the rehabilitation approach used for a tennis player should be unlike that used for a football player. However, often a re-habilitation specialist will be uncertain as to how a quarterback's rehabilitation program should differ from that of an offensive or defensive lineman. That is why your input is invaluable during functional progression, because coaches, like you, understand the demands placed on an athlete performing a certain activity.

BENEFITS OF FUNCTIONAL PROGRESSION

Let's look in more detail at the areas that functional progression serves as a positive tool in the care of the athlete. Functional progression is beneficial in that it

- promotes healing,
- provides a gauge of progress,
- establishes a bridge to participation,
- enhances self-confidence, and
- maximizes postinjury performance.

Promotes Healing

We have already discussed the important concepts in Wolff's and Davis's laws and the SAID principle. Healing tissue needs adequate force placed on it to facilitate optimal healing. These forces must be specific to the function that the involved tissue will assume when the athlete returns to full participation. Therefore, functional progression can help provide greater strength to healing tissue and yield a more thoroughly rehabilitated body part.

Provides a Gauge of Progress

In rehabilitation, muscle grades, muscle group ratios, and standard ROM parameters are used by rehabilitation specialists to gauge progress. However, although these standardized guidelines are beneficial in the clinic, they have no correlation to actual function on the athletic field.

Functional progression activities, when introduced properly, serve as useful tools for evaluating sport-specific function. A graduated program based on sport-specific activities serves as a "sport report card" that truly reflects the athlete's progress toward a return to competition.

Establishes a Bridge to Participation

Physical rehabilitation has been the focus of this section. However, functional progression also has psychological benefits. During rehabilitation, the athlete is removed from practice and game situations that bring enjoyment, comfort, and comaraderie. Therefore, the recuperating athlete may feel removed from his or her regular schedule and companions. Functional progression activities return the athlete to familiar surroundings and people with whom he or she feels comfortable.

Enhances Self-Confidence

During the course of rehabilitation, all athletes at one time or another ask themselves, Will I ever be able to perform like I could before my injury? This uncertainty is often warranted, especially when the athlete may be in danger of losing a spot on the starting team, a scholarship, or, in the case of a professional, a salary. This uncertainty may cause anxiety or apprehension. Pregame butterflies are normal, but excessive worry about function and reinjury can be minimized by a sound functional progression program.

After completing the ideal functional progression program, the athlete will not return to full competition without having been exposed to every possible situation that may be encountered during competition. If the athlete understands this, undue apprehension can be minimized.

Maximizes Postinjury Performance

Having gained from the four previously described benefits of functional progression, the athlete will reap one more advantage from this last step of sport rehabilitation: the ability to perform to his or her potential on returning to competition. This is in contrast to an athlete who hobbles and plays his or her way into shape and then becomes upset because of sub-par performance. With proper functional progression, your athlete and your team will go full speed ahead.

GUIDELINES FOR FUNCTIONAL PROGRESSION PROGRAMS

All injuries cannot be lumped together and rehabilitated in the same manner or in the same length of time. Thus, every injury must be handled on its own terms.

However, any functional progression program should conform to the following general guidelines:

- Functional progression should be introduced after formal rehabilitation.
- The activities should progress from simple to complex.
- The activities should be progressed only when tolerated.
- The athlete's performance must be closely monitored.

Functional Progression Introduced After Formal Rehabilitation

Adequate warm-ups, stretching, and any protective taping or equipment should precede functional progression. Prescribed therapeutic exercise should also be performed before attempting more vigorous activities.

Warm-up and stretching should always be the first thing an athlete does before working out. Then, therapeutic strengthening exercises that may possibly relax ligamentous tissue and tire muscle can be performed. Finally, the athlete can engage in activities that will optimally prepare him or her for practice and game participation.

Common sense, however, should dictate the functional progression regimen. In some cases, functional progression should precede strengthening or other activities to avoid negatively affecting the injured body part. Again, common sense suggests that the time to add highly stressful activity is not when the athlete is fatigued or at risk for reinjury. The athlete, the status of the injury, healing progress, and time constraints all must be considered during functional progression.

Activities Progressed From Simple to Complex

There should be no large leaps between steps in the functional progression program. Start with simple activities and progress to complex ones. For example, a basketball player's program should emphasize stationary jump shots before running, pull-up jump shots. In addition, functional activities should progress from slow to fast, easy to hard, and short to long.

Because most injuries occur in the late stages of practice or competition, functional progression activities usually should be performed after the athlete has worked out for some time. This approach more realistically simulates late-game and late-practice situations.

Activities Progressed Only When Tolerated

Steps in a functional progression program can be taken only if the previous step has been well tolerated. The athlete must not proceed to the next stage of functional progression if the athlete

- perceives instability in the involved area during performance,
- experiences pain during the activity,
- is overly anxious about performing the task,
- was unable to adequately complete the preceding task, or
- demonstrates pain, swelling, or decreased ROM following the previous task.

Performance Closely Monitored

Visual observation of the performing athlete and subsequent appropriate feedback are essential elements of functional progression. Filming the athlete is particularly beneficial because it permits performance to be analyzed in the presence of the athlete. After each step, it is wise to find out how the athlete felt or how he or she perceived function and to inspect the area for swelling. Prophylactic icing is a good idea after the workout.

FUNCTIONAL PROGRESSION TIME FRAMES

The amount of time required for healing must always be included in the sport rehabilitation program. The same holds true during the functional progression stage of the program. Thorough knowledge of time frames for healing is a prerequisite to effectively carry out the functional progression program.

Every injury is different, but specific injuries require a certain time period to heal. The sports medicine specialist knows these general time frames and, with the athlete and the coach, can prescribe activities in accordance with these time frames.

Sometimes, rehabilitation efforts cross the fine line between adequate stress that heals and strengthens tissues and too much stress that damages tissues. Activities that are excessive in frequency, duration, or intensity result in further tissue damage rather than tissue regeneration. Sometimes, rehabilitation efforts result in injury because the athlete attempts to return to action before the tissue is ready. Subpar ROM or strength also places excessive stress on injured tissue and predisposes it to reinjury. Therefore, a thorough understanding of the healing process and its time frames is necessary to conduct a functional progression program effectively.

As a rule, true functional progression does not begin until pain and swelling are gone. On the other hand, full AROM and adequate strength and endurance must be present.

A comprehensive sport rehabilitation program should not only include formal management of clinical symptoms such as pain, swelling, and weakness; it should also address functional concerns specific to each athlete's specific injury. This overlap of duties regarding formal injury management and functional progression highlights the need for a cohesive effort among the athlete, the coach, and the professional sports medicine specialist.

THE COACH'S ROLE IN FUNCTIONAL PROGRESSION

As mentioned at the beginning of this chapter, you have a vital role in this phase of your athletes' rehabilitation. Perhaps you have seen little room for your involvement in the rehabilitation process up to now because you felt that you had nothing to offer. But you, perhaps better than anyone on the sports medicine team, know the following:

- Each individual athlete on your team
- What can realistically be expected from that athlete
- How well the athlete must function to make a positive contribution
- The specific demands the athlete will face on a given play at a particular position
- When an athlete is using unnatural, substitute movements in performing a skill

Therefore, your active involvement is crucial to the success of the functional progression program. So get involved in the process and help your athletes return safely to competition by offering your expertise.

CONCLUSION

With an understanding of the basics of functional progression, you are now ready to look at some sport-specific approaches to functional progression.

The sports discussed in Appendices C, D, and E show how you can apply the functional progression principles discussed in this chapter. Remember, every injury is unique. And the examples used in these three appendices are only general guidelines and are not intended to represent a cookbook approach to all injuries sustained in a given sport. But with an understanding of functional progression and how a program can be designed that meets the specific demands of an athlete in your sport, you can become a more active participant in this last, vital stage of rehabilitation.

CHAPTER SUMMARY

1. After the clinical goals of stopping pain and swelling and achieving full ROM, adequate muscle strength, and sufficient endurance are satisfied, injury rehabilitation efforts turn to restoring the function that is necessary for the athlete to compete safely.
2. The graduated program of sport-specific drills that ready an athlete for a return to competition is called functional progression.
3. Physical benefits received by an athlete undergoing a functional progression program are the gradual stressing of injured tissue to make it stronger, a specific measurement tool to objectively measure function, and a sport-specific final test that bridges the gap between clinical rehabilitation and the playing field.
4. Psychologically, functional progression allows the athlete to interact with the coach and teammates in a familiar environment and enhances the athlete's self-confidence.
5. Functional progression should be progressed logically, timely, and only after prerequisite function is sufficient.
6. Your role is vital in this stage of rehabilitation. You are the expert who knows the demands placed on the athlete when he or she returns to competition. Your active input is absolutely necessary.

Part Summary

In this part, we explored the real nuts and bolts of sport rehabilitation. By discovering proper modes to improve your athletes' flexibility, strength, and proprioception, you will be better able to monitor your athletes' progress in the sport rehabilitation program. Many effective flexibility, strengthening, and proprioception exercises can be implemented into your athletes' training schedules.

A working knowledge of the supportive aids available to your athletes, above and beyond standard protective equipment, will also help you contribute to the sport rehabilitation process. Many of these additional protective devices can be easily fabricated with little expense.

Perhaps the most beneficial chapter of this part is the last one, which deals with functional progression. You are a key person during this essential and yet frequently overlooked part of the sport rehabilitation program. You should have a thorough knowledge of the demands that will be placed on your injured athletes on returning to competition, and your intimate involvement during this stage of the rehabilitation program should be your paramount concern.

Appendix A
Stretching Reference

Motion	Structures stretched	Substitutions
Shoulder flexion	Latissimus dorsi; posterior deltoid; posterior shoulder capsule; long head of triceps	Thoracic and lumbar spine extension (leaning backward)
Shoulder extension	Pectorals; anterior deltoid; long head of biceps; anterior shoulder capsule	Lumbar flexion (leaning forward)
Shoulder abduction	Pectoralis major; latissimus dorsi; inferior shoulder capsule	Lateral trunk flexion (away from the arm being abducted)
Shoulder external rotation	Anterior shoulder capsule; pectorals; latissimus dorsi	Thoracic and lumbar spine extension (leaning backward)
Shoulder internal rotation	Posterior shoulder capsule; teres minor; infraspinatus	Shoulder (scapular) protraction (rolling shoulders forward)
Shoulder horizontal adduction	Posterior shoulder capsule; posterior deltoid; middle trapezius; rhomboids; infraspinatus; teres major and minor	Lumbar and thoracic rotation (twisting trunk to opposite side)
Shoulder horizontal abduction	Anterior shoulder capsule; anterior deltoid; pectoralis major	Lumbar and thoracic rotation (twisting trunk to same side)
Elbow flexion	Triceps	
Elbow extension	Biceps; wrist flexors and extensors	
Wrist flexion	Extensor carpi radialis and ulnaris; common finger extensors	Elbow flexion
Wrist extension	Flexor carpi radialis and ulnaris; common finger flexors	Elbow flexion
Hip flexion	Gluteus maximus; hamstrings (upper); lumbar paravertebrals	
Hip extension	Rectus femoris; sartorius; iliopsoas	Lumbar flexion (leaning forward)
Hip adduction	Hip abductors (tensor fascia lata, gluteus minimus)	Lumbar flexion (leaning forward)
Hip abduction	Hip adductors (magnus, longus, brevis); gracilis	
Knee flexion	Quadriceps (vastus laterlis, vastus medialis, vastus intermedius, rectus femoris); sartorius	Lumbar flexion (leaning forward)
Knee extension	Hamstrings (semimembranosis, semitendinosis, biceps femoris)	Knee flexion; lumbar and thoracic flexion
Ankle dorsi flexion	Gastrocnemius; soleus	Plantar flexion; knee flexion

Appendix B
Therapeutic Exercise Reference

Structures	Conditions	Structures to stretch	Structures to strengthen
Cervical spine (upper trapezius)	Strain; brachial plexus stretch (burner, stinger)	Upper trapezius; pectorals	Upper trapezius; levator scapulae; sternocleido-mastoids; anterior neck flexors
Shoulder (anterior capsule)	Anterior subluxation or dislocation		Subscapularis; anterior deltoid; pectorals; supraspinatus; teres major
Supraspinatus tendon	Strain (tendinitis): impingement syndrome, swimmer's shoulder	Pectorals	Supraspinatus; teres major and minor; infraspinatus; rhomboids; middle trape-zius; serratus anterior
Acromioclavicular joint	Sprain (separated shoulder)		Pectorals; anterior deltoid
Biceps tendon (long head)	Strain (tendinitis)	Biceps; pectorals	Biceps (emphasize eccentric contractions)
Elbow (wrist extensors)	Strain (tendinitis): tennis elbow	Wrist extensors and supinators	Wrist extensors (empha-size eccentric contractions and grasp activities)
Wrist flexors	Strain (tendinitis)	Wrist flexors and pronators	Wrist flexors (emphasize eccentric contractions and grasp activities)
Hip (iliopsoas tendon)	Strain (tendinitis): snapping hip	Iliopsoas; rectus femoris	Iliopsoas (emphasize eccentric contractions)
Adductors	Groin strain	Adductors of hip	Adductors of hip; hip abductors (gluteus medius, iliotibial band)
Iliopsoas, rectus femoris	Groin strain	Hip flexors (rectus femoris, sartorius; iliopsoas)	Rectus femoris; sartorius; iliopsoas
Knee (patellar tendon)	Strain (tendinitis): patellar tendinitis, jumper's knee	Rectus femoris; sartorius; quadriceps femoris; hamstrings; calves	Quadriceps (emphasize eccentric contractions and hip extensors)

(Cont.)

Structures	Conditions	Structures to stretch	Structures to strengthen
Iliotibial band	Strain (tendinitis)	Hip abductors (iliotibial band, tensor fascia lata)	Tensor fascia lata
Patellofemoral joint	Patellofemoral pain; chondromalacia patellae (possible subluxation or dislocation)	Quadriceps; hamstrings, calves; iliotibial band	Quadriceps (especially vastus medialis)
Ankle (lateral ligaments)	Sprain	Calves	Anterior tibialis; ankle evertors
Ankle evertors	Strain	Calves	Anterior tibialis; ankle evertors
Achilles tendon	Strain (tendinitis)	Calves	Anterior tibialis; calves (emphasize eccentric contractions)
Anterior tibialis	Strain (tendinitis): anterior shin splints	Calves	Anterior tibialis; long-toe extensor
Posterior tibialis	Strain (tendinitis): posterior shin splints	Calves	Posterior tibialis (emphasize eccentric contractions); ankle evertors; anterior tibialis
Plantar fascia	Fasciitis	Calves; long-toe flexor	Toe flexors; anterior tibialis

Appendix C
Functional Progression for Football

Football players attempting to return to activity must progress through stages of function, depending on the type and site of the injury and the position played.

The following program should be introduced only if the injured athlete has

- no pain,
- no swelling,
- full ROM,
- adequate strength, and
- a normal walking pattern.

LOWER EXTREMITIES

The program outlined in Table C.1 is an effective approach to initiating efforts to restore sport-specific function to football players with lower extremity injuries.

Unloaded Activities

Functional progression activities for football must proceed from unloaded to loaded activities. Unloaded activities are performed by the athlete alone (no one else applies the resistance). Thus, the player performing unloaded activities can decrease or increase the inten-

**Table C.1
Functional Progression
for Lower Extremity Football Injuries**

Drills	Activities (unloaded)
1. Walk/jog/run program	Isolated team running

2. Step-ups
   Forward and backward
   Side to side
	Weight-lifting (squats, leg press)

3. Straight-plane jumping
   Forward and backward
   Side to side
   Diagonal
	Footwork drills (dummy chop-step crossovers); rope drills/tire drills

4. Straight-plane hopping
   Forward and backward
   Side to side
   Diagonal
	Half-speed 1-on-1 pass-rush drills

5. Agility drills
   Figure eights
   Carioca
   Straight-plane back-
     pedaling
	Speed-specific pass routes and shadow pass coverage

6. Cutting Forward and backward	Noncontact scrimmage

sity of participation according to his limitations. Loaded activities, on the other hand, involve two or more individuals applying resistance to one another.* Such activities

---

Note. These definitions of loaded and unloaded activities apply specifically to sport rehabilitation and should not be confused with the usage of these terms in other settings.

present a greater risk of injury (or reinjury) because the athlete cannot control the intensity of the force applied.

Walk/Jog/Run Program

Because football is primarily an anaerobic sport, jogging to ensure that the lower extremities can tolerate the forces of running should begin at a distance of a quarter mile. Distance should be increased in quarter mile increments until the athlete can jog 1 mile.

The emphasis of the program should be on anaerobic work in the form of sprints. Initial distances of 40 yards are adequate. The athlete should begin by jogging the first 10 yards, sprinting at half speed for the next 20 yards, and finishing with a 10-yard jog. As function improves, the middle 20 yards should be run at three-quarter speed and finally at a full sprint. When the athlete can sprint the middle 20 yards with little difficulty, the pace of the last 10 yards should be increased to half speed. Next, have the athlete sprint at three-quarter speed for the entire 40 yards. Finally, have the athlete perform full-speed 40-yard sprints. Defensive backs, offensive backs, and receivers should increase their full-speed-sprint distance to 100 yards.

Step-Ups

Step-ups are performed by having the athlete use the involved leg to step up onto an elevated surface. A platform can be built, or a stool, bleacher, or step can be used. The beginning height should be 4 to 6 inches and increased gradually as function improves.

The athlete should first step onto the elevated structure with the involved leg and then bring the uninvolved leg to the same height. The athlete should return to the floor by accepting weight on the involved side and then bringing the uninvolved leg down. This should be repeated as fast as possible *under control*. Three sets of 30 repetitions are adequate. The sequence is then repeated sideways as the athlete places the involved side nearest the step, raises up onto the step with the involved side, and then follows with the noninjured leg. The second set of 30 repetitions should be performed with the athlete facing the opposite way, leading with the uninvolved leg when stepping up but leading with the involved leg when descending.

Jumping and Hopping

Players who play positions that require jumping, such as receivers and defensive backs, will need another step in the functional progression program. Jumping and hopping allow the injured leg to accept greater forces, as body weight and momentum offer additional stress. Forward and backward jumping over a line painted on the floor can be progressed to side-to-side work and then diagonal jumping. Three sets of 30 jumps in each direction are appropriate. Jumping on both legs should be progressed to hopping on only the involved leg forward and backward, side to side, and then diagonally.

Figure Eights

Figure eights are important to ready the athlete for sharp cutting. The athlete should start with 10 40-yard figure eights at half speed, progress to three-quarter speed, and then finish at full speed. When the athlete masters these full-speed figure eights, cut the distance to 20 yards. Again, the athlete should progress from half-speed to three-quarter-speed and then to full-speed figure eights. After this sequence is completed, decrease the distance to 10 yards, using the same speed progression.

Agility drills and backpedaling can be started during this phase and be followed by cutting. The athlete should perform straight cuts, in which he plants the involved leg and cuts to the opposite side, and crossover cuts, in which he plants the involved leg and crosses the uninvolved leg in front and cuts to the side of the involved leg. The athlete should progress from half to three-quarter to full speed. Cutting should first be performed at a predetermined spot and then progressed to cutting on command. In specific injuries to the knee, cutting on command may be risky, so guidelines should be set by the rehabilitation specialist.

Loaded Activities

Once past this stage, the athlete should be able to perform any noncontact function. Progression should then be geared to load activities such as blocking and tackling (see Table C.2).

Head-On Blocking and Tackling

A 1-on-1 drill in which the athlete blocks and is blocked and another in which the athlete tackles and gets tackled should begin at half speed. These drills should be in a straight line (straight plane), with the injured athlete approaching his teammate head-on at half speed. You should emphasize proper blocking and tackling techniques. Speeds can be increased to three-quarter and then full speed.

Table C.2
Functional Progression
for Lower Extremity Football Injuries

Drills	Activities (loaded)
1. Resisted ball-carrying, blocking, and tackling drills	Dummy drills, sled work, and blaster drill
2. 1-on-1 straight-plane ball-carrying, blocking, and tackling drills	Head-up line play (5 yd)
3. 1-on-1 multiplane ball-carrying, blocking, and tackling drills	1-on-1 drills (10-20 yd)
4. Team-play, multiplane ball-carrying, blocking, and tackling drills	2-on-1 drills; 1-on-2 drills (10-20 yd); pursuit tackling (field as needed); special teams coverage

Multiplane Blocking and Tackling

Once full-speed head-on drills have been completed, the athlete can begin drills in which blocking and tackling angles are added (multiplane). Multiplane drills add the element of lateral movement and require pursuit, which involves accelerating or decelerating the basis of the actions of a teammate. Multiplane drill speeds begin at half speed and are gradually increased to three-quarter and then full speed. Finally, 2-on-1 drills involving blocking and being blocked, as well as tackling and being tackled, can be added. Again, the athlete

should participate on the side that double-teams and also receive the double-team. The next step is scrimmage and then full practice drills.

Kicking

Skill positions, such as placekickers and punters, should emphasize specific skills. Once stationary kicking and punting motions are pain free, the athlete can begin taking steps before kicking. Punters may use a half-speed stepping approach to the punting position. Early in the functional progression program, a lighter ball (e.g., high-density foam rubber) may be used if necessary. Proper kicking and punting mechanics rather than distance should be emphasized. Distances half of what is normal for the athlete should be the initial goal. Approach speeds may then be increased to normal, and the athlete can begin kicking farther until normal distance is achieved. After these activities can be performed without difficulty in isolated practice, the kicker and punter may then take part in scrimmage sessions and then game situations.

UPPER EXTREMITIES

Upper extremity functional progression is required for a football player to support body weight in a down position and to block, tackle, and fall.

Unloaded Activities

As in the lower extremity functional progression, activities should progress from unloaded to loaded. Unloaded activities should begin with weight bearing on both arms. Activities such as a four-point position, bear crawls, push-ups, and other drills are appropriate. Once tolerated, these activities can be advanced by having the athlete perform wheelbarrow drills. Table C.3 provides a step-by-step outline of upper extremity drills and activities to use with your football players.

Wheelbarrow Drill

This drill is similar to the old wheelbarrow races except that the athlete's arms must do

Table C.3
Functional Progression
for Upper Extremity Football Injuries

Drills	Activities (unloaded)
1. Bilateral support drills	Bear crawl; up-and-downs
2. Unilateral support drills	Spinning wheelbarrows; arm hopping

3. Controlled falling
  Forward roll
  Shoulder roll (forward and backward)
  Tumbling
	Small-group drills (e.g., monkey-roll drill)

the work of the wheel. Initially at half speed for 10 yards, this drill should progress in 10-yard increments up to 30 yards. The distance is then reduced to 10 yards at three-quarter speed and increased to 20 and then 30 yards. Finally, these distances can be covered at full speed.

Roll Drills

Because football involves falling, controlled falling in the form of forward rolls (somersaults) should be emphasized in the functional progression program. Somersaults place weight on the shoulder girdle. As the athlete tucks his chin and rolls forward, the weight is accepted between the shoulder blades. Starting from a squat, forward and backward somersaults should be progressed to forward rolls from half-speed to three-quarter-speed to full-speed runs. Forward rolls are then replaced by stationary forward and backward shoulder rolls. This drill involves bearing weight directly on the shoulder. Once stationary shoulder rolls are performed easily, the athlete can execute rolls from a half-speed run. The football player should eventually progress to three-quarter-speed and full-speed running shoulder rolls.

Spinning Wheelbarrow

Another good way to isolate single-arm weight bearing is to have the athlete place the hand

of the involved arm flat on the ground. Using this arm as a pivot, the athlete now spins around the fixed arm in clockwise and counterclockwise directions. The athlete can progress by increasing the number of circles in each direction and increasing the speed in which he pivots around the fixed arm.

Arm Hopping

Arm hopping incorporates additional weight bearing on the arm and is the next step in the functional progression. Arm hopping involves the same structures as those used in pivoting arm circles. However, in this case the athlete runs at half speed to a predetermined spot on the field and then, with hips and knees bent, places the involved arm down to the ground. From this three-point stance, the athlete pushes off the arm, propels himself up to a running position, and continues down field. Arm hopping can be started at a distance of 30 to 40 yards with an arm hop every three strides. The athlete should increase his pace to a three-quarter-speed run and then to full speed. Distances can be increased from 30 to 60 yards and finally to 100 yards.

Loaded Activities

Once unloaded drills have been completed, the athlete can begin loaded contact drills (see Table C.4). The football player must be able to deliver and accept forces through the injured upper extremity. Drills that involve bilateral delivery and acceptance of forces should be emphasized and progressed to actions involving the injured side only.

Blocking and Pass Rushing

Offensive and defensive linemen can begin 1-on-1 pass blocking or pass-rushing drills. Speed should be progressed from half speed to three-quarter speed to full speed. The emphasis in performing the drills should be placed on proper technique and body position. These activities should initially be head-on and then progress to angle line play. After 1-on-1 drills have been mastered, 2-on-2 drills can be added and progressed in a manner similar to that for lower extremity injury.

Table C.4
Functional Progression
for Upper Extremity Football Injuries

Drills	Activities (loaded)
1. Bilateral force delivery and acceptance	Pass blocking; defensive shivers
2. Unilateral force delivery and acceptance	1-on-1 tackling and blocking; line play (5, 10, and 20 yd); pursuit (field as needed); special teams coverage

Pass Receiving

Skill positions such as pass receivers should emphasize specific skills (e.g., pass catching) to allow for a complete return to competition. Initially, a lightweight ball can be used if necessary. The receiver should then catch low-velocity passes from short distances. The velocity of the passes in these drills should increase gradually from half speed to three-quarter speed to full speed. After two-handed catching is performed with little difficulty, isolating the involved upper extremity for single-handed pass catching can also be beneficial.

Passing

A quarterback with an upper extremity injury should engage in a return-to-passing program (see Table C.5). Again, a lightweight ball may be used, and proper throwing mechanics should be emphasized. The quarterback should begin by throwing 8 to 10 yards for 5 minutes. Keeping the distance the same, he can increase throwing time every other day by 5 minutes. Early in the program, the athlete should rest the day after passing.

Once the athlete is up to 15 minutes of 8- to 10-yard passing at half speed, he can increase the velocity to three-quarter speed. The first and last 3 to 4 minutes should involve passing at half speed to warm up and cool down and the middle 7 to 9 minutes passing at three-quarter speed. The middle 7 to 9 minutes can later be increased to 10 to 15

Table C.5
Return-to-Passing Program
for Upper Extremity Football Injuries

1. Stationary short toss (8-10 yd)
   _____ 50% velocity
   _____ 75% velocity
   _____ 100% velocity
2. Stationary intermediate toss (10-20 yd)
   _____ 50% velocity
   _____ 75% velocity
   _____ 100% velocity
3. Shotgun set (live throwing)

8-10-yd patterns	10-20-yd patterns
_____ Simple	_____ Simple
_____ Advanced	_____ Advanced

4. Drop-back pass (live throwing)

8-10-yd patterns	10-20-yd patterns
_____ Simple	_____ Simple
_____ Advanced	_____ Advanced

5. Rollout pass (toward involved side)

8-10-yd patterns	10-20-yd patterns
_____ Simple	_____ Simple
_____ Advanced	_____ Advanced

6. Rollout pass (toward uninvolved side)

8-10-yd patterns	10-20-yd patterns
_____ Simple	_____ Simple
_____ Advanced	_____ Advanced

7. Stationary long toss
   30-50-yd patterns
   _____ Simple
   _____ Advanced

Note. Simple patterns include hooks, look-ins, and short crossing routes. Advanced patterns include timing, deep fly, and down-and-out patterns.

minutes, bringing the total passing time up to 18 to 20 minutes. At this point, the quarterback's passing velocity can be increased to full speed using the same progression. Finally, throwing distance can be increased to 10 to 20 yards.

The next step in the quarterback's functional progression is to take snaps from the center and throw to receivers running pass patterns. Because the shotgun precludes much of the drop-back movement and thus provides a more stable base from which to throw, the quarterback should begin with this offensive set. Pass routes should be kept short and simple and progress in difficulty. Once the athlete has performed these activities with no difficulty, he can begin drop-back passing. The progression of throws should follow that described for the shotgun phase. When drop-backs are performed without difficulty, roll-outs can be added, first rolling out to the involved side and then to the uninvolved side. Finally, long pass routes can be added.

Appendix D
Functional Progression for Volleyball

Volleyball players jump and strike the ball forcefully. Thus, both the lower and the upper extremities of these athletes must be fully functional before an injured athlete can return to competition. And because many movements in basketball parallel those made in volleyball, you can easily adapt much of this volleyball program to the needs of your basketball players.

The following program should be introduced only if the athlete has

- no pain,
- no swelling,
- full ROM,
- adequate strength,
- sufficient endurance, and
- a normal walking pattern.

LOWER EXTREMITIES

Because quick and powerful lateral and vertical movements are required for volleyball participation, the lower extremities must be fully functional before a player is allowed to return to competition. The following activities are effective for achieving such sport-specific function (see Table D.1).

Table D.1
Functional Progression for Lower Extremity Volleyball Injuries

Drills	Activities
1. Walk/jog/run program	Isolated team running

2. Step-ups
  Forward and backward
  Side to side
	Reaching on toes at net; stationary setting; serving; bumping

3. Straight-plane jumping
  Forward and backward
  Side to side
  Diagonal
	Stationary jumping drills at net; lateral slide drills

4. Straight-plane hopping
  Forward and backward
  Side to side
  Diagonal
	Lateral jumping drills at net; stationary spiking drills

5. Agility drills
  Figure eights
  Carioca
	Full-speed approach of net; spiking, setting, and bumping; jump serves

6. Cutting Forward and backward	Scrimmage

Walk/Jog/Run Program

Because volleyball is chiefly an anaerobic sport, emphasis should be placed on quick burst sprints. However, to ensure lower extremity tolerance of running and to build an aerobic base, the athlete should begin jogging up to 1 mile and increase distance by quarter-mile increments. Anaerobic sprints of no greater than 30 to 40 yards should also be performed. A sprinting progression similar to the one described in Appendix C is recommended.

Step-Ups

Step-ups can be performed and progressed as described in Appendix C (p. 132). However, because volleyball demands much more jumping than football, a greater emphasis should be placed on step-ups by athletes in this sport. For example, an appropriate step-up workout might include two or three bouts of three 30-repetition sets. Care must be taken not to aggravate or create problems in extensor mechanisms (quadriceps, quadriceps tendon, patella, and patellar tendon).

Jumping and Hopping

Jumping on both legs and hopping on the involved leg helps the legs accept the stress created by momentum plus body weight. Initially, three 30-jump repetitions can be attempted at the net to reestablish blocking skills. Another option for this drill is to have the athlete jump for three 1-minute bouts with a 1-minute rest between sets. The volleyball player should emphasize quick, explosive movements.

The athlete can progress from these repetitive jumps from a stationary position to hopping on the involved leg only. These single-leg drills should include three sets of 15 repetitions or three 30-second bouts with a 1-minute rest between sets.

Simple plyometrics (e.g., jumping on and off a bench with both legs), if tolerated, can be performed when jumping and hopping drills are no longer difficult. Excellent texts devoted to plyometrics, such as *Plyometrics: Explosive Power Training* by Radcliffe and Farentinos, are available. A weighted belt, weighted vest, or resistive tubing can be used to make jumping and hopping drills even more strenuous.

Agility Drills and Cutting

The figure-eight progression described in Appendix C (p. 132) should be performed so that the athlete can accommodate rotational and torsional stresses. These activities should be progressed from half speed to three-quarter speed to full speed. And full-court figure eights should be progressed to half the length of the court.

Straight cuts and crossover cuts, first at the predetermined site and then on verbal or visual command, should be progressed from half to three-quarter to full speed (refer to Appendix C). Because volleyball requires short, quick lateral movements as well as stops and pivots, your athletes should mimic those actions in mirror drills. The players should start and stop quickly, pivot forward and backward, and move side to side and diagonally. Speeds of the drills should be progressed from half to three-quarter to full speed.

UPPER EXTREMITIES

Emphasis in upper extremity functional progression for volleyball is tailored to the postures that players must assume to produce or absorb forces (see Table D.2).

Proper form should be the primary emphasis, especially when athletes perform overhead motions. Serving motions without a ball can be introduced, and, when function is not compromised or painful, resistance can be added. An effective form of resistance for serving is a foam rubber ball.

Bumping, blocking, serving, spiking, and setting drills can also begin. When these activities have been successfully completed with lightweight resistance, the regulation volleyball can then be added.

Blocking, bumping, and digging should be initiated from short distances, and the speed of the incoming ball should be slow. Three 30-second bouts can begin with the ball hit to the athlete at half speed. Speeds can be increased to three-quarter and then to full speed. These activities should progress from the ball coming straight to the athlete to shots that require the athlete to react to the ball side to side, front and back, and at angles.

Table D.2
Functional Progression
for Upper Extremity Volleyball Injuries

Drills	Activities
1. Overhead form drills	Shadow-serving, spiking, and setting drills

2. Controlled falling
    Forward roll
    Shoulder roll (forward and backward)
    Tumbling
	Shoulder rolls after dig

3. Bilateral force-absorption drills	Light to heavy blocking, digging, and bumping
4. Bilateral force-delivery drills	Light to heavy blocking and setting
5. Unilateral force-absorption drills	Involved upper extremity digs
6. Unilateral force-delivery drills	Light to heavy serving, hitting, and spiking

Initial serving and spiking efforts should emphasize putting the ball in play at a desired location. Serves should be performed for 5 minutes initially and increased by 5 minutes every other day until the player is serving for a total of 15 to 20 minutes. Serving velocity should progress from half to three-quarter to full speed. Spiking should begin from a slow-paced set from you or a teammate and progress to spiking a returned ball from the opposite side of the net. Again, the speed of the spikes should increase from half to three-quarter to full speed.

Because volleyball also involves contact with the floor when digging and diving for the ball, players should include such activities in the program. The forward rolls and shoulder rolls described in Appendix C (p. 134) are certainly appropriate for this part of the volleyball functional progression program. But before the player returns to competition, repeated practice digs and dives from a variety of spots on the floor must be performed effectively and without pain.

Appendix E

Functional Progression for Baseball and Softball

Once again, before introducing the following program with an athlete, make sure the player has

- no pain,
- no swelling,
- full ROM,
- adequate muscle strength,
- sufficient endurance, and
- a normal walking pattern.

LOWER EXTREMITIES

Too often in the rehabilitation of baseball and softball players, the functioning of the athlete's arm is considered more important than the legs. But these two sports demand numerous lower extremity functions (e.g., pushing off the mound, sprinting out of the batter's box, sliding into a base) that can be performed only by a functionally sound athlete. The program outlined in Table E.1 will help an athlete achieve these functions.

Walk/Jog/Run Program

Because baseball is a sport of quick sprints and quick reactions, your program should emphasize anaerobic work. When the player can jog 1 mile with no swelling, pain, or dysfunction,

**Table E.1
Functional Progression for Lower Extremity Baseball and Softball Injuries**

Drills	Activities
1. Walk/jog/run program	Outfield running; playing catch; pepper games (hitting only)
2. Step-ups Forward and backward Side to side	Batting practice
3. Straight-plane jumping and hopping Forward and backward Side to side Diagonal	Controlled infield and outfield drills (no cutting or pivoting)
4. Figure eights, cutting, and baserunning	Full-speed infield and outfield drills; stealing, sliding, and baserunning; noncontact double-play drill
5. Special skills	Pitching and catching

you can introduce a vigorous sprinting program into the athlete's regimen. Start the athlete on the right-field foul line at medium depth (slightly further than halfway between the edge of the infield dirt and the outfield fence). The athlete should jog at half speed for

30 feet and then sprint at half speed across the outfield toward a similar position down the left-field line. The athlete should slow down to a half-speed jog for the final 30 feet. When the player is ready to progress, the half-speed sprint can be increased to three-quarter speed and then full speed. Once this presents no difficulty, the athlete can begin the sprint from a stationary start, first at half speed, then at three-quarter speed, and finally at full speed.

Step-Ups, Jumping, and Hopping

Jumping and hopping (e.g., footwork on a double play) is sometimes required in defensive situations. To ensure that the athlete can accept full body weight without problems, the player should perform three sets of 10 to 15 repetitions of forward and side step-ups (forward and backward and side to side) and diagonal jumping and hopping.

Figure Eights

Again, these drills are a prerequisite to cutting. The athlete should begin at home plate and run a figure-eight pattern to shallow center field and back. Half-, three-quarter-, and full-speed figure eights should be performed at this distance. Then the distance can be decreased from home to second base and finally from home to the pitcher's mound. Speed can be increased as just described. Three sets of 10 repetitions are adequate.

Cutting

A cutting sequence can be made more functional for baseball players by including baserunning drills. However, straight cuts and crossover cuts should be performed (see Appendix C, p. 132) before more difficult baserunning maneuvers. Then the player should attempt to push off a base with the involved leg. Half-, three-quarter-, and full-speed baserunning drills that include these movements should be performed.

Although baseball is typically thought of as a noncontact sport, high-risk positions (catcher, second baseman, and shortstop) may want to gradually prepare for contact. Collisions at home plate or second base are not necessary; however, the athlete should engage in agility drills that approximate the body positions used to avoid contact.

UPPER EXTREMITIES

Overuse upper extremity injuries are common in baseball and softball. Acute arm injuries occur less frequently. Once the throwing arm is injured, a carefully progressed return-to-throwing program (see Table E.2) is necessary to help ensure the athlete's complete recovery and safe return to competition.

Lob-Toss Program

Initial throwing distances should be sufficient to allow a normal overhand throwing motion without "short-arming" the ball. The athlete should be able to throw the ball in a normal fashion, emphasizing follow-through. Depending on the level of play, distances between 20 and 60 feet may be appropriate.

If the athlete is able to concentrate on form and not worry about overthrowing, a foam rubber ball may be used initially. Again, the player should emphasize form more than distance. Velocities should be kept low (half speed) when a baseball or softball is used. One way to regulate throwing speed is to prohibit athletes from using a glove while they play catch. Initial bouts of throwing are usually limited to 5 to 10 minutes or 60 to 120 throws at half speed. The athlete should rest the arm the day after throwing. Each subsequent throwing session should be increased by 5 minutes unless the athlete experiences pain or swelling. After throwing for 20 minutes, the athlete can increase velocity from three-quarter to full speed.

Any decrease in velocity, loss of ball control, or pain experienced during throwing indicates that additional strengthening and functional progression efforts are required before additional throwing is allowed.

Table E.2
Return-to-Throwing Program for Baseball and Softball

Activities	Duration	Distance

1. Lob-toss program
    Bare-handed catch
    Foam rubber balls
	5-10 min	10-20 ft

2. Half-speed throwing	5-10 min or 60-120 throws	20-60 ft increasing to 60-90 ft
3. Outfield throwing program	5-10 min or 60-120 throws	Medium-deep center field increasing to deep center field
4. Full-speed throwing	15-20 min	From regular playing position
5. Additional pitcher and catcher work		

Once the player can throw full speed for 20 minutes without difficulty, the distance can be increased to 60 to 90 feet. Velocity at this distance should be half speed before timely increases to three-quarter and then full speed.

To develop greater arm strength, the throwing program is then moved to the outfield. The recuperating athlete should assume a position in medium-deep center field. From there, the athlete should throw the ball to second base on a roll. Ten minutes of this long tossing is followed with the short-throwing program of 60 to 90 feet. Later, the athlete should throw the ball into second base on one hop. Again, 10 minutes of this activity should be followed by short-distance (60 to 90 feet) throwing. Finally, the athlete is allowed to throw the ball to second base on a fly.

When the athlete can throw to second base on a fly, the distance is increased as the player moves into deep center field. The program is repeated from this position.

After full-speed, deep-center-field throws are performed easily, outfielders can work on reaching the cutoff person and progress to throwing all the way to each base (progressing from closest to farthest). For example, the right fielder should throw to second base before throwing to third base.

Infielders can then resume their positions on the infield and take part in infield practice drills. Once back in the infield, the athlete should throw while moving toward the base to which the ball is being thrown. When ball velocity and accuracy are appropriate, the player can begin throwing while moving away from the base to which the ball is being thrown (e.g., shortstop fielding a ball between short-stop and third base and attempting to throw to first base).

Catchers should be able to throw to the pitcher without difficulty at this stage. When beginning to throw to second base, the catcher should throw from a standing position. Only after getting the ball to second base with normal velocity and accuracy should the catcher attempt to throw to second after receiving a pitched ball. Velocity progression during these stages should be from half to three-quarter to full speed.

After completing the long-toss program in the outfield, pitchers should begin working off the mound. A full windup should be used, and the pitcher should concentrate on proper form while throwing fastballs only. When normal

Table E.3
Simulated-Game Guidelines
for Baseball and Softball

1. Warm-up	Throw for 10-15 min and gradually increase velocity (total of 50-80 pitches). Then throw 5-10 pitches to warm up before beginning each inning.
2. Game performance	Throw the number of innings usually required per outing based on level of play, league rules, and starter versus reliever (professional pitcher averages 5-8 innings, 12-18 pitches per inning).
3. Rest	Rest approximately 9 min between innings.

velocity and control are attained, progression is made to throwing breaking balls (curves and sliders).

Pitchers and catchers will benefit from simulated games, such as the one outlined in Table E.3. However, the averages listed in this table were obtained from studies of professional games. Therefore, you may wish to alter your simulated games to a more appropriate level.

Glossary

accessory motion—An involuntary, non-physiological motion necessary for normal range of motion

active-assisted range of motion (AAROM)—Active range of motion that is assisted through all or part of the normal range of motion

active range of motion (AROM)—Range of motion that is performed voluntarily

acute fracture—A macrotraumatic injury that disrupts normal bone continuity

acute phase—The first 48 to 72 hours after macrotrauma, marked by a loss of active range of motion and strength

aerobic—Requires the presence of oxygen

agonist—A muscle that works in conjunction with other muscles to promote movement

anaerobic—Does not require the presence of oxygen

antagonist—A muscle that works against and restricts the movement of an agonist

atrophy—A decrease in muscle size resulting from disuse

blanching—The whitening of an area after manual pressure is removed following cryotherapy

brachial plexus stretch—A traction or stretch injury of the cervical nerve roots (C5-T1), usually occurring from excessive lateral flexion of the neck. Also called burner, stinger

burner—*See* brachial plexus stretch

bursa—A fluid-filled sack located between two tissue layers that decreases friction between the tissues

bursitis—An inflammation of a bursa

chondromalacia patellae—A wearing away or softening of the kneecap's articular surface

chronic phase—A period beginning no earlier than 6 months after macrotraumatic injury in which the injury remains unresolved or reinjury occurs

collagen—The connective tissue protein in ligaments and tendons

concentric—A muscle contraction in which muscle fibers shorten and move the muscle insertion toward the muscle origin

conduction—The therapeutic heat produced by an exchange of energy from one object to another

continuous ultrasound—The therapeutic heat produced by continuous ultrasound waves

contraction—The shortening of a muscle or muscle fiber

contraindication—A condition with which specific therapeutic measures should not be performed

convection—The production of therapeutic heat from movement of the heating medium

conversion—The therapeutic heat produced by transferring one energy form into another

cryotherapy—The therapeutic application of cold or ice

dislocation—A joint injury that forces apart the bones comprising a joint, thereby disrupting the joint capsule

eccentric—A muscle contraction that lengthens the muscle fibers and causes the muscle insertion to distance itself from the muscle origin

elasticity—The physical property of collagen that allows muscle tissue to stretch and then return to its original length

electromyography—The study of electrical current generated in muscle tissue

endorphines—The opiates that are produced naturally in the central nervous system

fracture—A break in bone continuity

functional electrical stimulation (FES)—The use of therapeutic electrical current to generate muscle contraction

functional progression—A graduated series of sport-related activities that prepares a previously injured athlete to return to sport

goniometer—A device used to measure range of motion

high-voltage galvanic stimulation (HVGS) An electrotherapeutic modality that increases or decreases local circulation and/or stimulates muscle contraction

hip pointer—A contusion of the pelvic iliac crest

Hunting reflex—The name given to vasodilation that is claimed to occur after prolonged cold applications

hydrocollator—A commercially available heating unit that maintains water at a constant temperature to store hydrocollator packs

hydrocollator pack—A gel pack that is stored in hot water and is used to deliver moist heat

internal joint derangement—A nonspecific diagnosis indicating that problems exist within a joint

interstitial space—The space separating two cell walls

iontophoresis—The use of electrical current to deliver anesthetic or anti-inflammatory agents to an injured area

isokinetic—Muscle work that applies resistance to the muscle at a predetermined, constant rate throughout a joint's range of motion

isometric—Muscle action that has no subsequent joint motion

isotonic—Muscle work that applies constant resistance to the muscle

lateral epicondylitis—An inflammation of the origin of the wrist and finger extensors

lymphatic system—The system that filters venous blood

macrotrauma—An injury sustained from a single, nonrepetitive event

mechanoreceptors—Receptors located in joints that provide stimulus information to the brain

medial elbow overload—Stress of the soft tissues in the medial elbow that usually results from an excessive valgus angle

medial epicondylitis—An inflammation of the muscular origin of the wrist and finger flexors

microamperage electrical nerve stimulation (MENS)—The therapeutic use of milliamperage electrical current

microtrauma—An injury sustained from repetitive events

modality—A therapeutic medium including any one of a variety of technologies or physical means to aid in injury rehabilitation

myelin—A soft white insulating sheath surrounding certain nerve fibers

myofascial pain syndrome—A clinical diagnosis characterized by trigger points with tight muscles and/or referred pain

myositis ossificans—An abnormal calcification of extracellular blood in muscle tissue

nociceptors—Nerve endings that are responsible for sending sensations of pain to the brain

opiate—A derivative of opium that has a pain-reducing effect

orthotic—Any external device that is applied to the body to augment normal function

osteochondritis dissecans (OCD)—A complete or partial separation of joint cartilage from the underlying bone

osteoporosis—The loss of bone density

overload principle—Loading a muscle to the point of fatigue and progressing that load as tolerated

passive range of motion (PROM)—Range of motion that is performed involuntarily

phonophoresis—Delivering anesthetic or anti-inflammatory preparations to an injured area with ultrasound

physiological motion—Range of motion that can be performed voluntarily

plantar fascia—A thick, fibrous band located on the bottom of the foot that provides support to the arch

plantar fasciitis—An inflammation of the plantar fascia

plexus—An area where nerves and/or blood vessels meet

precaution—A condition in which specific therapeutic measures should be used only with caution

prepatellar bursitis—An inflammation of the prepatella bursa

prime mover—A muscle or group of muscles responsible for a given physiologic motion

proprioception—The sensory awareness of body joint position resulting from signals sent to the brain

pulsed ultrasound—Automatically cycled ultrasound waves that are used therapeutically to increase circulation and do so with less heat than continuous ultrasound

quad set—An isometric contraction of the quadricep muscles

range of motion (ROM)—The normal movement parameters of a given joint

reciprocal innervation—Nerve fibers that allow a muscle to produce smooth joint movement by contracting and relaxing

secondary hypoxic injury—An injury to tissue from decreased blood supply

secondary mover—A muscle or group of muscles that assist prime movers in physiological motion

sprain—An injury to ligamentous tissue.

stinger—*See* brachial plexus stretch

strain—An injury to muscle or tendinous tissue

stress fracture—A microtraumatic injury that disrupts bone continuity by an excessive breakdown of bone

subacute phase—The period following the acute phase (the first 48 to 72 hours after injury) and possibly continuing for 6 to 12 months, in which pain and swelling are diminished and motion and strength are increased

subluxation—A joint injury that forces the structures of the joint partially apart without disrupting the joint capsule

swelling—The abnormal enlargement of an injury site from excess fluid build-up

tendinitis—An overuse injury that results in inflamed muscle tendons

traction apophysitis—The inflammation of an independent growth center, or apophysis, caused by muscle pulling on it

transcutaneous electrical nerve stimulation (TENS)—The therapeutic application of a portable device that generates electrical current to decrease pain

vasoconstriction—The narrowing of blood vessel circumference

vasodilation—The widening of blood vessel circumference

venous system—The vascular system that returns blood to the heart from peripheral body parts

viscoelasticity—Property of being both elastic and viscous; used to describe tissues

Suggested Reading List

Alter, M. (1988). *Science of stretching*. Champaign, IL: Human Kinetics.

American Academy of Orthopaedic Surgeons. (1985). *Knee braces seminar report*. Chicago: Author.

American Academy of Orthopaedic Surgeons. (1987). *A position statement: The use of knee braces*. Chicago: Author.

Baker, B., Vanhanswyk, E., Bogosian, S., Werner, F., & Murphy, D. (1987). A biomechanical study of the static stabilizing effect of knee braces on medial stability. *American Journal of Sports Medicine*, **15**, 566-570.

Bergeron, J.D. (1989). *Sport injuries study guide*. Champaign, IL: Human Kinetics.

Bergeron, J.D., & Greene, H.W. (1989). *Coaches guide to sport injuries*. Champaign, IL: Human Kinetics.

Bunch, R., Bednarski, K., Holland, D., & Macinanti, R. (1985). Ankle joint support: A comparison of reusable lace-on braces with traditional taping and wrapping. *The Physician and Sportsmedicine*, **13**(5), 59-62.

Coleman, A., Axe, M., & Andrews, J. (1987). Performance profile-directed simulated game: An objective functional evaluation for baseball pitchers. *Journal of Orthopaedic and Sports Physical Therapy*, **9**, 101-105.

Cooper, D., & Fair, J. (1979). Contrast baths and pressure treatment for ankle sprains. *The Physician and Sportsmedicine*, **7**, 143.

Curwin, S., & Stanish, W. (1984). *Tendinitis: Its etiology and treatment*. Nova Scotia: D.C. Heath.

France, E., Paulos, L., Jayaraman, G., & Rosenberg, T. (1987). The biomechanics of lateral knee bracing. Part 2: Impact response of the braced knee. *American Journal of Sports Medicine*, **15**, 430-438.

Garrick, J., & Regua, R. (1987). Prophylactic knee bracing. *American Journal of Sports Medicine*, **15**, 471-476.

Glick, J., Gordon, R., & Nishimoto, D. (1976). The prevention and treatment of ankle injuries. *American Journal of Sports Medicine*, **4**, 136-141.

Gould, J., & Davies, G. (Eds.) (1985). *Orthopaedic and sports physical therapy*. St. Louis: C.V. Mosby.

Grace, T., Skipper, B., Newberry, J., Nelson, M., Sweetster, E., & Rothman, B. (1988). Prophylactic knee braces and injury to the lower extremity. *Journal of Bone and Joint Surgery*, **70**(A), 422-427.

Harvey, J. (Ed.) (1985). Rehabilitation of the injured athlete. *Clinics in Sports Medicine*, **4**, 405-583.

Hewson, G., Mendini, R., & Wang, J. (1986). Prophylactic knee bracing in college football. *American Journal of Sports Medicine*, **14**, 262-266.

Hughes, L. (1983). A comparison of ankle taping and a semirigid support. *The Physician and Sportsmedicine*, **11**, 99-103.

Jackson, D. (1984). The history of sports medicine: Part 2. *American Journal of Sports Medicine*, **12**, 255-257.

Jackson, D., Ashley, R., & Powell, J. (1974). Ankle sprains in young athletes. *Clinical Orthopaedics and Related Research*, **101**, 201-215.

Kegerreis, S. (1983). The construction and implementation of functional progression as a component of athletic rehabilitation. *Journal of Orthopaedic and Sports Physical Therapy*, **5**, 14-19.

Kegerreis, S., Malone, T., & McCarroll, J. (1984). Functional progressions: An aid to athletic rehabilitation. *The Physician and Sportsmedicine*, **12**(12), 67-71.

Keggerreis, S., & Wetherald, T. (1987). The utilization of functional progressions in the rehabilitation of injured wrestlers. *Athletic Training*, **22**, 32-35.

Knight, K. (1985). *Cryotherapy: Theory, technique, and physiology.* Chattanooga, TN: Chattanooga Corporation Educational Division.

Paulos, L., France, E., Rosenberg, T., Jayaraman, G., Abbott, P., & Jaen, J. (1987). The biomechanics of lateral knee bracing. Part I. Response of the valgus restraints to loading. *American Journal of Sports Medicine*, **15**, 419-429.

Radcliffe, J.C., & Farentinos, R.C. (1985). *Plyometrics: Explosive power training* (2nd ed.). Champaign, IL: Leisure Press.

Rovere, G., Haupt, H., & Yates, S. (1987). Prophylactic knee bracing in college football. *American Journal of Sports Medicine*, **15**, 111-116.

Roy, S., & Irvin, R. (1983). *Sports medicine: Prevention, evaluation, management, and rehabilitation.* Englewood Cliffs, NJ: Prentice-Hall.

Smith, R., & Reischl, S. (1986). Treatment of ankle sprains in young athletes. *American Journal of Sports Medicine*, **14**, 465-471.

Snook, G. (1984). The history of sports medicine: Part 1. *American Journal of Sports Medicine*, **12**, 252-253.

Teitz, C. Hermanson, B., Kronmal, R., & Diehr, P. (1987). Evaluation of the use of braces to prevent injury to the knee in collegiate football players. *Journal of Bone and Joint Surgery*, **69**(A) 2-8.

Tropp, H., Askling, C., & Gillquist, J. (1985). Prevention of ankle sprains. *American Journal of Sports Medicine*, **13**, 259-261.

Vaes, P., DeBoeck, H., Handelberg, F., & Opdecam, P. (1985). Comparative radiologic study of the influence of ankle joint bandages on ankle stability. *American Journal of Sports Medicine*, **13**, 46-50.

Wilkerson, G. (1985). External compression for controlling traumatic edema. *The Physician and Sportsmedicine*, **13**, 97-106.

Wilkerson, G. (1985). Treatment of ankle sprains with external compression and early mobilization. *The Physician and Sportsmedicine*, **13**(6) 83-96.

Yamamoto, S., Hartman, C., Feagin, J., & Kimball, G. (1975). Functional rehabilitation of the knee: A preliminary study. *American Journal of Sports Medicine*, **3**, 288-291.

Zachezewski, J. (1986). Flexibility for the runner: Specific program considerations. *Topics in Acute Care and Trauma Rehabilitation*, **2**, 9-27.

Index

A

Abrasion, 20
Accessory motion, 68
ACEP (American Coaching Effectiveness Program)
    Sport First Aid and Sport Injuries, 5
Acetic acid, 61
Achilles tendinitis, 87, 103, 120, 130
Achilles tendon rupture, 80, 97
Active-assisted range of motion (AAROM), 68
Active range of motion (AROM), 67
Acute postinjury phase, 27, 75
Aerobic fitness, 35
Agonist, 69, 73
Allied health specialists, 11
American Academy of Sports Medicine Physicians, 8
American College of Sports Medicine, 13-14
American Dietetic Association, 13
American Physical Therapy Association, 12, 14
Anaerobic fitness, 36
Ankle sprain, classification of, 26
Anorexia nervosa, 13
Antagonist, 69, 73
Aorta, 41
Arteries, 41
Arterioles, 41
Aspirin, 60
Association for the Advancement of Applied Sport
    Psychology, 14
Athletic trainer, 11-12

B

BAPS (biomechanical ankle platform system) board, 107
Baseball
    common injuries in, 23
    functional progression for, 141-144
    simulated game of, 143
    throwing injuries, 23
Basketball, common injuries in, 122-124
Biofeedback, 104
Blanching, 44
Blazina classification, of overuse injuries, 28
Body movement
    description of, 68
    planes of, 68
Brachial plexus stretch, 22, 101, 114, 129
Bracing after sport injury, 112
Bradykinin, 27
Bulimia, 13
Burner. *See* Brachial plexus stretch
Bursa, 21
Bursitis, 21

C

Cable tensiometer, 92
Capillaries, 26, 41
Cardiac disorders, cryotherapy and, 45

Cardiologist, 8
Cardiovascular conditioning
    aerobic, 36
    anaerobic, 35
    lack of, 35
    with rehabilitation program, 95
Carpals, 25
Cerebellum, 106
Cervical spine
    injuries to, 21
    muscles of, 22-23
Chondromalacia patellae. *See* Patellofemoral pain
Chronic injury phase, 27, 75
Circulation
    abnormal, 41, 45
    decreasing, 41-42
    increasing, 52-53
    normal, 41
Clavicle, 23-24
Coach
    functional progression and the, 121, 125
    limitations in sport rehabilitation, 4
    responsibilities in sport rehabilitation, 3, 19
    safety measures and the, 32
    training methods and the, 32-33
Cold hypersensitivity, 45
Cold spray, topical application of, 58
Cold therapy. *See* Cryotherapy
Collagen, mechanical properties of, 69-70
Communication, 4
Compression, 43
    application of, 45-47
    constant, to decrease swelling, 41, 45
    intermittent, to decrease swelling, 47
Conform (brand of adhesive tape), 113
Contrast baths, 58
Contusion, 20
    of ankle, 58
    of brachialis, 83
    of elbow, 58
    of thigh, 116-117
Coracoacromial ligament, 23-24
Cortisol, 56
CPR (cardiopulmonary resuscitation), 4
Cryokinetics, 44
Cryotherapy, 41, 95
    application of, 43-44
    common indications for, 45
    decreasing pain with, 58
    physiological effects of, 42
    precautions and contraindications for, 45
    versus compression, 43

D

Dancers, common injuries of, 21
Davis's law, 121

Dead-arm syndrome, 109
Deconditioning, 35
Deep heating modalities, 53
Dentist, 8
Dermatologist, 8
Dexamethasone, 61
Dietician
    duties and responsibilities, 12-13
    education and training, 13
    employment setting, 12-13
Dislocation, 20, 24
Dynamometer
    hand-held, 92
    isokinetic, 91-92

E

Eccentrics. *See* Muscle contraction, eccentric
Ectomorph, 75
Edema. *See* Swelling
Elastic bandages, 45
    application of, 46
    common widths used for specific injuries, 46
Elasticity, 70, 74
Elasticon (brand of adhesive tape), 113
Electrical current, bodily effects of, 48, 61
Electrical stimulation
    to decrease swelling, 41, 47-48
    to increase muscle strength. *See* Functional
        electrical stimulation (FES)
Electroacupuncture, 59-60
Electromyography, 94
EMG. *See* Electromyography
Endogenous opiate theory of pain relief, 59
Endorphins, 59
Ensolite, 112
Erythema, 44
Ethyl chloride, 58
Exercise. *See also* Exercise to improve proprioception;
        Exercise to increase range of motion; Exercise to
        increase strength
    guidelines, 77
    resistance
        isokinetic, 91, 94, 104
        isotonic, 91, 94, 104
        surgical tubing and, 98, 100
        Theraband and, 99-101
Exercise physiologist
    duties and responsibilities, 13
    education and training, 13
    employment setting, 13
Exercise to improve proprioception, 105
    after ankle injury, 107
    after knee injury, 108-109
    after shoulder injury, 109
Exercise to increase range of motion
    of calf, ankle, and foot
        acute phase, 80-81
        chronic phase, 87
        subacute phase, 83
    of cervical spine
        acute phase, 77
        chronic phase, 84
        subacute phase, 82
    of elbow, wrist, and hand
        acute phase, 78
        chronic phase, 85-86
        subacute phase, 82-83

    of hip, pelvis, and groin
        acute phase, 79-80
        chronic phase, 86
        subacute phase, 83
    of knee
        acute phase, 79-80
        chronic phase, 86-87
        subacute phase, 83
    of shoulder
        acute phase, 77
        chronic phase, 84-85
        subacute phase, 82
    of upper, lower back
        acute phase, 78
        chronic phase, 86
        subacute phase, 83
Exercise to increase strength, 89, 95
    acute phase, 96-97
    of calf, ankle, and foot
        acute phase, 97
        chronic phase, 103-104
        subacute phase, 100-101
    of cervical spine
        acute phase, 96
        chronic phase, 101
        subacute phase, 97-98
    chronic phase, 101-104
    of elbow, wrist, and hand
        acute phase, 96
        chronic phase, 101-102
        subacute phase, 98
    of hip, pelvis, and groin
        acute phase, 96-97
        chronic phase, 102
        subacute phase, 99
    of knee
        acute phase, 97
        chronic phase, 103
        subacute phase, 100
    of lower back
        acute phase, 96
        chronic phase, 102
        subacute phase, 100-101
    of shoulder
        acute phase, 96
        chronic phase, 101
        subacute phase, 101
    subacute phase, 97-100
Extracellular space. *See* Interstitial space

F

Femur, 25
Fibula, 25
First aid, 4-5
Flat neck posture, 84
Fluoromethane, 58
Football, common injuries in, 21, 24-25, 98, 117
    functional progression, 131-136
Forward head posture, 84
Forward shoulder posture, 85
Fracture, 20
Functional electrical stimulation (FES)
    application of, 95
    indications for, 94-95
Functional progression, 37, 65, 95, 121
    baseball, 141-144
    benefits of using a, 122-123

football, 131-136
guidelines for, 123-124
precautions, 124
softball, 141-144
volleyball, 137-139

G

Gate control theory of pain relief, 59
General practitioner, 8
Glenohumeral joint
dislocation, 20, 24, 78, 82, 96, 101, 109, 114-115, 129
subluxation, 20, 78, 82, 96, 101, 109, 114-115, 129
Goals
of *Coaches Guide to Sport Rehabilitation*, vii
of sport rehabilitation, 33-37
Goal setting in sport rehabilitation
short-term, 31-32
long-term, 31-32
Gymnastics, common injuries in, 21, 109

H

Heat production, 52
Hemarthrosis, 72
High voltage galvanic stimulation (HVGS), 47-48
application of, 48
indications for, 47
precautions and contraindications for, 48
Hip pointer, 79, 116
Histamine, 26-27, 42, 45
Hockey, common injuries in, 21
Hot packs. *See* Hydrocollator packs
Humerus, 23
Hunting reflex, 42
Hydrocollator, 53
Hydrocollator packs
application, 53
description, 53
indications for, 53-54
Hydrocortisone, 60
Hydrotherapy
description, 54
indications for, 54-55
precautions and contraindications, 55
temperatures of, 54-55
treating open wounds, 55
Hypermobility, 75
Hypertonicity, 73

I

Ice bags, 43
Ice massage, 44
Ice packs, 43-44
Ice water immersion, 58
Imagery, 13
Immobilization
and abnormal range of motion, 73-74
effects of, 33, 35, 94, 113
Impingement syndrome, 23, 82, 84, 96, 101, 129
Inflammation, 27, 42, 52, 54-55, 60
Internal joint derangement, 72
Interstitial space, 26, 41
Interval training, 36
Intervertebral foramen, 21
Iontophoresis
application, 61
precautions and contraindications, 61
Ischemia, 27

J

J Flex (brand of adhesive tape), 113
Joint mobilization, 69
Jumpers, common injuries of, 27
Jumper's knee, 34, 103, 129

K

Knee bracing, 118-119

L

Labral tear (shoulder), 73
Laceration, 20
Lacrosse, common injuries in, 21
Lateral epicondylitis, 2, 85, 102, 115, 129
Laws of healing, 121
Legal limitations, of coaches, 4
Lidocaine, 60
Line jumping, 36
Lower extremity
bones of, 25
cardiovascular training after injury to, 36
joints of, 25
Lymphatic system, 41

M

Macrotrauma, 20, 29
Manual muscle test, 92
Manual resisted exercise, 94
Mechanoreceptors, 105, 110
Medial elbow overload, 25, 85, 102
Medial epicondylitis, 24, 85
Meniscal injury (knee), 72, 103
MENS. *See* Microamperage electrical nerve stimulation (MENS)
Metatarsals, 25
Microamperage electrical nerve stimulation (MENS)
application of, 61
indications for, 62
Microtrauma
definition of, 21
injury classification for, 28-29
Modalities. *See* Therapeutic modalities
Moleskin (adhesive tape), 113
Motivation, 13
Muscle
atrophy, 35, 72, 93
balance, 34
endurance, 33-34
extensor carpi radialis brevis, 24
extensor digitorum communis, 24
fibers, 93
function, 33
length, 34
calf, 34
hamstrings, 34
spasm, 52, 96
strain, 27
weakness, 35
Muscle contraction
concentric, 90, 91, 104
to decrease swelling, 49
eccentric, 90, 91, 94, 102-104
electrical stimulation and, 94-95
isometric, 96, 97, 104
Muscle strength, 33
assessment, 92

Muscle strength (*continued*)
benefits of, 89
grades, 94
Myofascial pain, 85
Myositis ossificans, 83

N

National Athletic Trainers' Association, 12, 14
National Strength and Conditioning Association, 14
Navicular fracture, 83, 86
Neoprene sleeve, 114-117
Nerve fibers
A fibers, 57, 59
C fibers, 57, 59-60
Neurologist, 8-9
Neurosurgeon, 9
Nociceptors, 57
North American Society for Psychology of Sport and
Physical Activity, 14

O

Ophthalmologist, 9
Opiates, 59
Oral surgeon, 9
Orofit, 115
Orthopedist, 8
Orthoplast, 112, 114-116, 118-119
Orthotic, 9, 120
Orthotist, 116
Osgood-Schlatter's disease, 21, 34, 103, 117
Osteochondritis dissecans (OCD), 21
Osteoporosis, 35
Otolaryngologist, 9
Overload principle, 90
Overstretching, 75
Overuse injury. *See* Microtrauma

P

Pain, 33, 52, 96, 101
experience and relief of, 57
medication to decrease, 57-58, 60-61
restricting range of motion, 72
Pain-spasm-ischemia cycle, 27, 39, 53
Paraffin baths, 54
Participation
criteria for resumption of, 36
time frames for, 36
Patellar tendinitis, 34, 103, 129
Patellofemoral joint
dislocation, 20, 100, 118, 130
subluxation, 20, 100, 118, 130
Patellofemoral pain, 34, 86, 103, 118, 130
Pediatrician, 8
Phonophoresis
allergic reactions to, 60
indications, 60, 62
precautions and contraindications, 60
Phoresor, 61
Physical therapist, 12
Physiologic motion, 68
Pivot shift, 108, 118
Plantar fasciitis, 26, 87, 103, 120, 130
Plantar warts, 56
Plasticity, 70
Plastizote, 112
Plyometrics, 103
Podiatrist, 9

Positive thinking, 13
Postinjury phases, 27
PPT padding, 115-120
Prepatellar bursitis, 118
Preseason screening, 33
Pressure dressings, used to decrease swelling, 45-47
Preventing sport injury, 31-33
PRICE (protection, rest, ice, compression, elevation)
system of injury management, 27-28, 31
Prime mover, 33, 69, 73
Proprioception, 35, 105, 110
assessing, 105-107
improving
ankle, 107
knee, 108-109
shoulder, 109
Protective devices, padding, and supports, 37, 111-114
after ankle injury, 119-120
after elbow, wrist, and hand injury, 115
after hip, groin, and pelvis injury, 116-117
after knee injury, 117-119
after low back injury, 116
after shoulder injury, 114-115
Protein, concentration in blood plasma, 41, 42

R

Radius, 23
Range of motion, 34
abnormal restrictions, 70-71
acute phase, 72-74
chronic phase, 83-84
subacute phase, 81-82
determining factors, 67
gravity-assisted, 67, 95
gravity-eliminated, 67, 95, 97
gravity-resisted, 67
passive, 68
principles of, 69
Raynaud's disease, 45
Reflex inhibition, 33, 72
Relaxation, 13
Rugby
common injuries, 21, 114
regarding protective padding, 113
Rule changes, affecting injury rates, 25
Runners, common injuries of, 21, 86

S

Safety measures, coach's role in providing for, 32
SAID (specific adaptations to imposed demands)
principle, 122
Scapula, 23, 25
Secondary hypoxic injury, 42
Secondary mover, 69, 83
Serotonin, 27
Sever's disease, 21, 87, 120
Shin splints, 130
anterior, 87
Shoulder dislocation. *See* Glenohumeral joint
Shoulder girdle, bones of, 24
Shoulder separation. *See* Sprain, acromioclavicular
Snapping hip, 86, 129
Sodium salicylates, 61
Spondylolysis (stress fracture of the back), 86
Sport injury
assessment, 29
classification, 20

coach's role in assessing, 28-29, 31
  defined, 19
  diagnosing, 19
  intervention in, 27
Sport psychologist, 13
Sport rehabilitation
  facilities, 5
  goals, 75
  personnel, 5
  program components, 31
  program implementation, 31-32
Sports medicine physician
  educational background, 7
  specialization areas, 8-9
Sports medicine specialist
  allied health professional, 11-14
  physician, 7, 9
  role, 7
Sprain
  acromioclavicular, 24, 82, 96, 114, 129
  ankle, 25, 81, 97, 100
  anterior cruciate ligament, 25, 72, 97, 100, 103,
    108, 118
  classification, 20
  medial collateral ligament (knee), 26
  posterior cruciate ligament, 103
  sternoclavicular, 114
Stationary cycling, 36
Step-ups, 36
Stinger. *See* Brachial plexus stretch
Strain
  calf, 81
  classification, 20
  factors contributing to a, 26
  groin, 26, 79, 97, 102, 129
  hamstring, 26, 100
  hip flexor, 97, 99, 102, 116, 129
  quadricep, 26
Strength and conditioning coach, 14
Strengthening
  ankle dorsiflexors, 100
  ankle evertors, 100
  deltoid, 101
  forearm pronators, 102
  forearm supinators, 102
  gluteus maximus, 99
  guidelines for common knee conditions, 103
  guidelines for success, 95
  hamstrings, 100
  levator scapula, 101
  pectoralis major, 101
  quadriceps, 100
  serratus anterior, 102
  sternocleidomastoid, 101
  trapezius (upper), 101
  wrist extensors, 102
  wrist flexors, 102
Strength training
  adjuncts to, 94-95
  duration, 93
  form, 93
  frequency, 93
  overtraining and, 93
  progression, 93-94
  recovery time, 93
Stress fracture of the back, 86

Stress management, 13
Stretching
  calves, 88
  force, 74
  hamstrings, 86
  iliotibial band, 87
  muscle temperature and, 75
  pectorals, 85
  program development, 74, 76
  quadriceps, 87
  reference, 127
  static versus ballistic, 74-75
  velocity, 74-75
Subacute injury phase, 27, 75
Subluxation, 20
Superficial heating modalities, 53-55
Supplemental readings, 3
Swelling, 41
  causes of, 26
  healing effects of, 27
  restricting range of motion, 72
Swimmers, common injuries for, 23

T
Tape
  after sport injury, 113
  application, 46
  to decrease swelling, 45
  types of, 46
Tarsals, 25
Tendinitis
  Achilles, 21
  biceps, 23
  iliopsoas, 26
  iliotibial band, 87, 129
  lateral epicondyle, 24
  medial epicondyle, 24
  patellar, 26
  supraspinatus. *See* Impingement syndrome
Tennis elbow. *See* Lateral epicondylitis
Tennis leg. *See* Strain, calf
TENS. *See* Transcutaneous electrical nerve stimulation
  (TENS)
Therapeutic heat
  depth of penetration, 51
  effect on peripheral versus core temperature, 51
  general versus local application, 51
  generation of, 52
  physiologic effects, 52-53
  precautions and contraindications, 51
Therapeutic modalities
  to decrease pain and inflammation, 57
  to decrease swelling, 41
  to increase circulation, 51
  in sport rehabilitation, 62
Tibia, 25
Tissue response to injury, 26
Traction apophysitis, 21
Training heart rate, 35
Training methods, coach's role in providing for, 32-33
Transcutaneous electrical nerve stimulation (TENS), 58
  application, 58-59
  development of, 58
  indications, 59
  pain relief afforded by, 59
  precautions and contraindications, 59
Trigger point, 85

U

Ulna, 23
Ultrasound, 55-56
Unhappy Triad of O'Donoghue, 119
Universal weight equipment, 98, 101
Upper extremity
   bones of, 23
   cardiovascular training after injury to, 36
   injuries to, 23

V

Vasoconstriction, 42, 48
Vasodilation, 42
Venous system, 41
Viscoelasticity, 70

Viscolas, 112
Volleyball
   common injuries, 23
   functional progression, 137-139

W

Warm-up, 95
Weight loss and gain, 13
Whirlpool. *See* Hydrotherapy
Wobble board, 106
Wolff's law, 121
Wrestling, common injuries in, 109, 118

X

Xylocaine, 61

About the Author

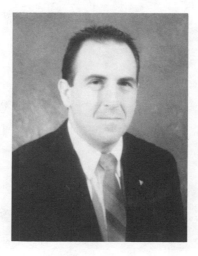

THE LEARNING CENTRE
HAMMERSMITH AND WEST
LONDON COLLEGE
GLIDDON ROAD
LONDON W14 9BL
0181 741 1688

Steven R. Tippett is undoubtedly one of the most experienced and qualified people to write on the topic of sport rehabilitation. In addition to being a certified athletic trainer, a certified physical therapist, a noted researcher, a national lecturer, and sports medicine and physical therapy instructor, Tippett's credentials include the following:

- 11 years of experience in the rehabilitation of musculoskeletal disorders,
- teaching sports medicine and orthopedic physical therapy at the university level,
- lecturing with nationally recognized physical therapists,
- being one of the original 16 physical therapists in the country certified by the American Board of Physical Therapy Specialties as a Sports Physical Therapist,
- being chosen by the US Olympic Committee to train the sports medicine staff of the Pan American Games
- assisting in a research project to examine the effects of strength training on the prepubescent athlete, and

Tippett is currently the Sports Medicine Director at St. Francis Hospital in Peoria, IL, where he works with injured athletes, athletic trainers, and sports medicine physicians on a daily basis.

In his spare time, Tippett enjoys spending time with his wife and their two children, writing sports medicine articles and case studies, and jogging.